The Complete Liver Cirrhosis Diet Cookbook For Seniors 2025

Beyond the Plate: Delicious Recipes, Lifestyle Strategies, and Essential Guidance for Thriving with Liver Cirrhosis

Seraphina Mercer

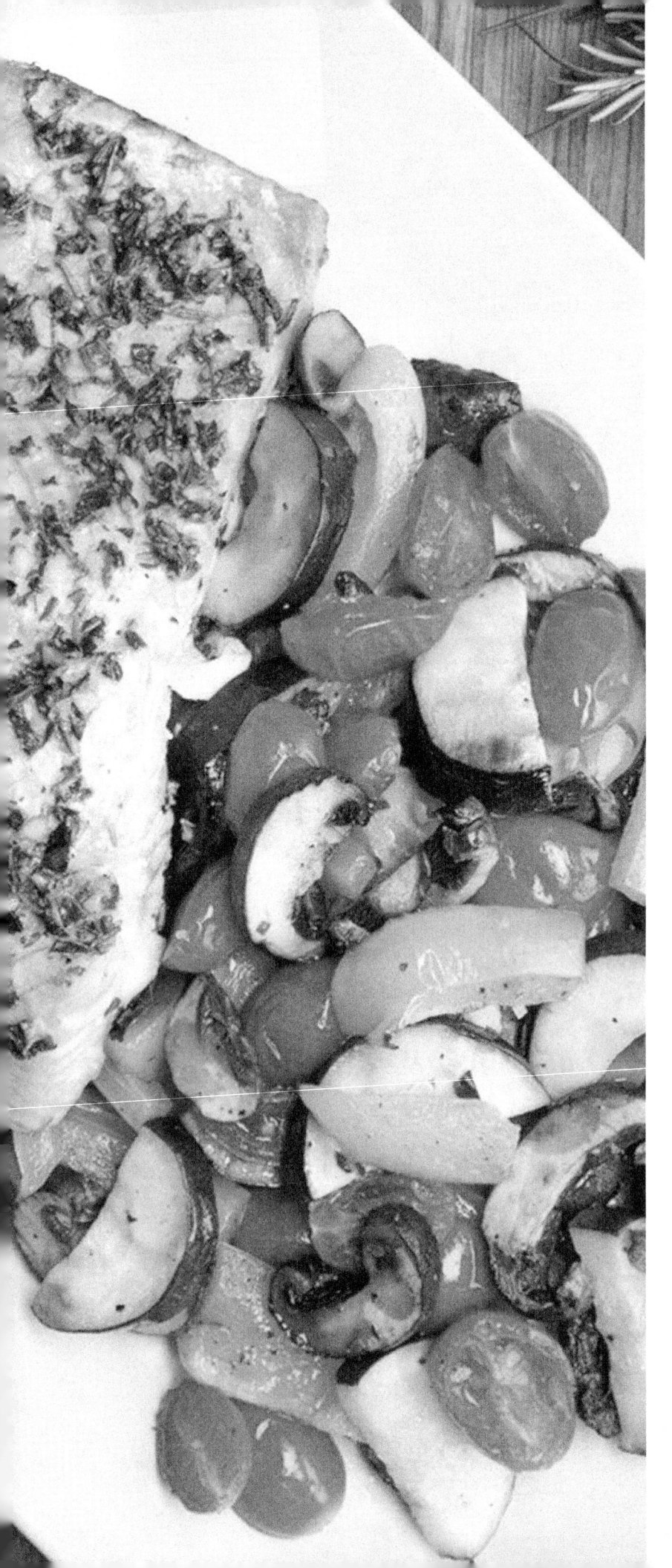

Copyright © 2025 Seraphina Mercer

All rights reserved. This publication may not be reproduced, distributed, or transmitted in any form or by any means—electronic, mechanical, photocopying, recording, or otherwise—without prior written consent from the publisher. The only exceptions permitted under copyright law are brief quotations in critical reviews and certain other non-commercial uses.

TABLE OF CONTENTS

- INTRODUCTION 2
- UNDERSTANDING LIVER CIRRHOSIS 5
- FOODS TO EMBRACE AND FOODS TO AVOID 8
- ESSENTIAL INGREDIENTS & KITCHEN TIPS 11
- BREAKFAST 14
- LUNCH 36
- DINNER 59
- SNACKS 79
- DRINKS 93
- SIDE DISHES 108
- LIFESTYLE TIPS FOR MANAGING LIVER CIRRHOSIS 109
- MEAL PLAN & SHOPPING LIST 123
- CONCLUSION 135
- BONUS 139
- INDEX 140

INTRODUCTION

Welcome. You've been told to change the way you eat. You've been told it's serious. You've been given a list of foods to avoid and little else. That's where most people start. Confused. Overwhelmed. Tired.

I'm a clinical dietitian. I've worked with seniors managing liver cirrhosis for over 15 years. I've seen the frustration. I've seen the fear. I've also seen what works.

One of my patients, Robert, was 72 when he was diagnosed. He lived alone. He didn't cook. He thought he had to give up everything he liked. For weeks, he ate plain rice and boiled chicken. His weight dropped. His energy tanked. He told me, "I'm doing everything right, and I feel worse."

We worked together. We kept things simple. We found ingredients that supported his liver. We built meals he could prepare in 15 minutes. We talked about snacks that didn't spike his sodium. In six weeks, he was cooking for himself again. He told me, "I feel like me again."

This book is based on what I've learned from patients like Robert. It's not about perfection. It's about patterns. Small changes. Meals that are gentle on your liver and easy on your energy.

You're here. That's a good start. Let's move forward.

Why This Cookbook?

This cookbook is designed for seniors with liver cirrhosis. It speaks directly to your needs, not general advice meant for everyone.

Liver disease changes how your body handles food. Your liver filters toxins, stores nutrients, and processes proteins. When it's damaged, everything shifts. What you eat matters more. What you avoid matters even more.

Older adults face added challenges:

- Slower metabolism
- Lower appetite
- Muscle loss
- Medication interactions
- Fatigue that makes cooking harder

This book addresses those issues with:

- Simple, nutrient-dense recipes
- Low-sodium, low-fat meals that protect liver function
- High-protein options to prevent muscle loss
- Easy instructions for limited energy days
- Ingredient swaps to cut risk without cutting taste

Each recipe supports your liver. Each section answers a question you're likely asking.

This isn't just a cookbook. It's a tool. A guide to eating with purpose. A way to make meals safer without making them bland.

You won't find miracle cures. You'll find real food. Real strategies. Built for your body and your stage of life.

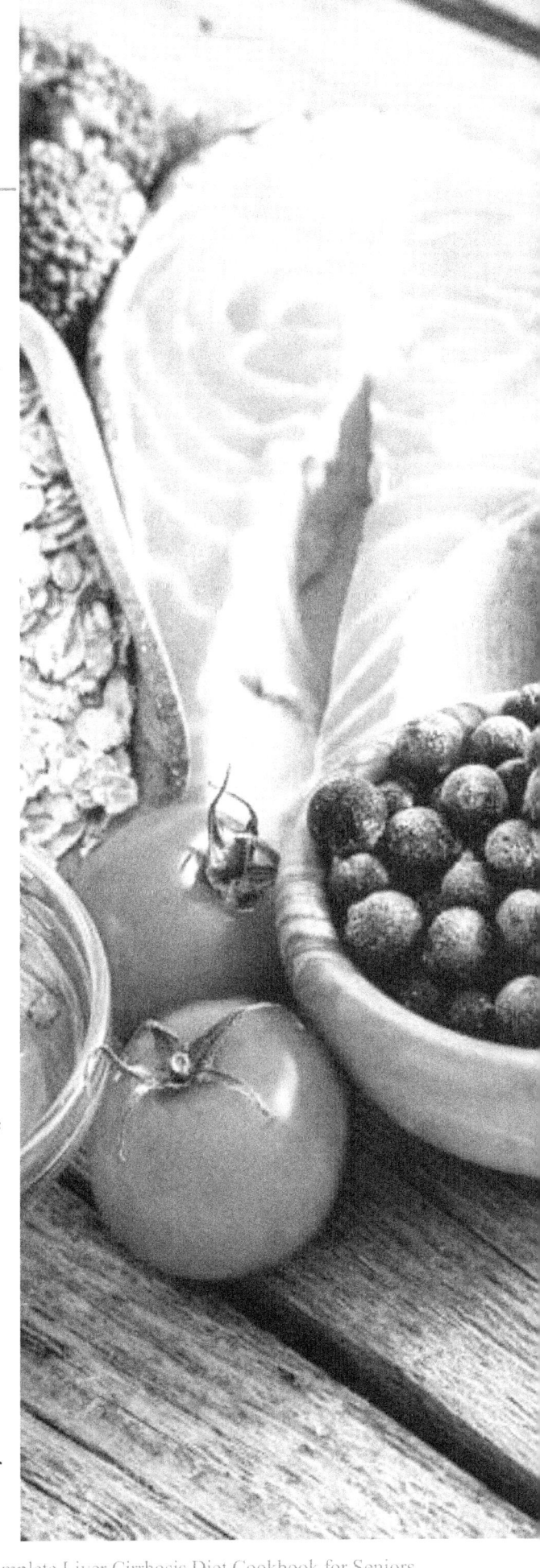

The Emotional Impact of Liver Disease

Liver disease doesn't just affect the body. It affects how you feel, how you think, and how you connect with others. Many seniors with cirrhosis report anxiety. You worry about the future. About symptoms. About hospital visits. You feel uncertain about every bite you take.

Depression is common. Loss of appetite, fatigue, and disrupted sleep can lower your mood. You might feel frustrated or hopeless. Simple tasks feel harder. Food loses its appeal. You lose interest in things you once enjoyed.

Some patients isolate themselves. They avoid family dinners. They turn down invitations. They feel like a burden. They're tired of explaining their condition. Tired of saying "no" to food. Tired of pretending they feel fine.

One patient, Margaret, said, "I stopped going to church potlucks. I didn't want to answer questions. I didn't want people to feel sorry for me." Social withdrawal creates a cycle. Less connection leads to more depression. Less support makes it harder to follow a diet. It becomes a lonely struggle.

This book helps break that cycle.

Food is social. Sharing meals builds connection. Safe, liver-friendly meals help restore confidence. They allow you to say "yes" again—to breakfast with your daughter, to coffee with a friend, to life. You're not your diagnosis. You still have choices. You still have tools.

Let food be one of them.

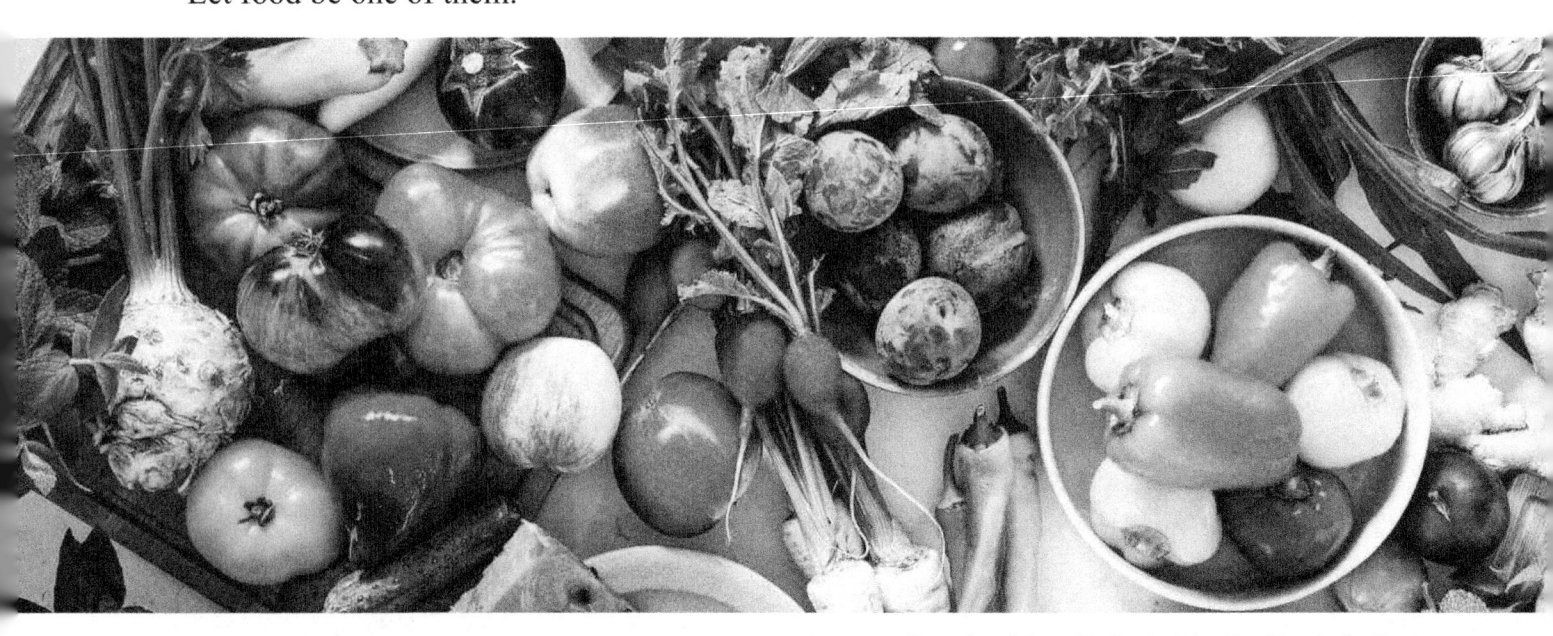

CHAPTER 01

UNDERSTANDING LIVER CIRRHOSIS

What is Liver Cirrhosis?

Liver cirrhosis is long-term damage to the liver. It replaces healthy tissue with scar tissue. This scar tissue blocks blood flow and weakens the liver's function.

Your liver filters toxins, makes proteins, and stores nutrients. When it's scarred, it struggles to do those jobs. Damage builds slowly, often over years.

Common Causes

- Chronic hepatitis B or C
- Long-term alcohol use
- Fatty liver disease (linked to obesity and diabetes)
- Autoimmune liver conditions
- Certain medications and toxins
- Genetic disorders (like hemochromatosis)

Symptoms

- Fatigue
- Loss of appetite
- Nausea
- Swelling in legs or belly
- Yellowing of skin or eyes (jaundice)
- Confusion or memory trouble
- Bruising easily

How Diet Helps:

Your liver processes everything you eat. A poor diet makes its job harder. The right diet reduces stress on your liver and helps manage symptoms.

Key goals:

- Control sodium to reduce swelling
- Support protein needs without straining digestion
- Avoid alcohol and added sugars
- Choose healthy fats over saturated fats
- Get enough vitamins and minerals from whole foods

Essential Nutrients for Liver Health

Your liver works every minute. It breaks down food, removes toxins, and stores energy. When it's damaged, it needs help. That help starts with nutrients.

Key Nutrients Needed for Liver Health

Protein

- Helps prevent muscle loss, common in cirrhosis
- Supports tissue repair and immune function
- **Choose lean sources:** eggs, fish, poultry, legumes
- Spread intake through the day to ease digestion

Sodium (Keep It Low)

- High sodium causes fluid buildup in the legs and belly
- Aim for less than 2,000 mg per day
- Skip canned soups, processed meats, frozen meals
- Use herbs, garlic, and lemon for flavor

Healthy Fats

- Your liver handles fat poorly when damaged
- Avoid fried foods, butter, and red meat fat
- Use small amounts of olive oil or avocado
- Eat nuts, seeds, and oily fish in moderation

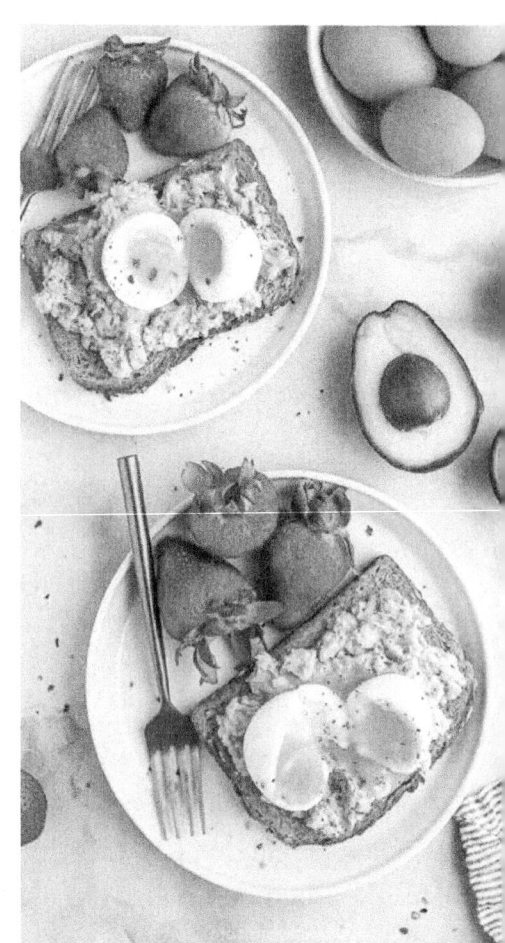

Vitamins and Minerals

- Cirrhosis affects nutrient absorption
- You may need more:
    - **Vitamin D**: supports bones and immunity
    - **Vitamin A**: low in liver disease, but avoid excess
    - **Zinc**: helps with protein use and appetite
    - **Magnesium**: supports muscle and nerve health
    - **B vitamins**: support energy and brain function

Hydration and Its Importance for Cirrhosis Management

Your liver needs water to function. Without enough fluid, your blood thickens. Toxins build up. Digestion slows. Dehydration puts stress on every part of your system—including your liver.

Why Hydration Matters:

- Helps the liver flush waste
- Supports digestion and bowel regularity
- Prevents fatigue and confusion
- Reduces risk of kidney strain, common in cirrhosis

Practical Tips:

- Drink small amounts throughout the day
- Keep water by your bed and chair
- Set reminders to sip every hour
- Flavor water with lemon or cucumber
- Eat high-water foods: melon, cucumber, broth, soup
- Use a straw if swallowing is hard
- Limit drinks that dehydrate: coffee, soda, alcohol

Aim for 6 to 8 cups per day unless your doctor says otherwise. In late-stage cirrhosis, fluid limits may apply—follow medical advice.

CHAPTER 02

FOODS TO EMBRACE AND FOODS TO AVOID

Liver-Supporting Foods

The right foods help your liver do its job. They reduce inflammation. They support healing. They make digestion easier. These are foods to include often.

Vegetables

- Broccoli, spinach, carrots, kale, beets
- High in fiber and antioxidants
- Help the liver filter toxins
- Steam or roast with olive oil

Fruits

- Apples, berries, oranges, bananas, grapes
- Rich in vitamins and fiber
- Support digestion and reduce inflammation
- Choose whole fruits over juice

Whole Grains

- Brown rice, oats, quinoa, barley
- Provide slow-burning energy
- High in fiber for digestive health
- Avoid added salt or seasoning packets

Lean Proteins

- Chicken, turkey, fish, eggs, tofu
- Needed to maintain muscle
- Easier to digest than red meat
- Bake, grill, or poach

Legumes

- Lentils, chickpeas, black beans
- High in plant protein and fiber
- Support steady blood sugar
- Rinse canned beans to lower sodium

Healthy Fats

- Avocados, olive oil, flaxseeds, walnuts
- Contain omega-3 fatty acids
- Reduce liver inflammation
- Use in small amounts

Low-Fat Dairy

- Yogurt, milk, cottage cheese
- Source of calcium and protein
- Choose unsweetened, low-sodium options

Herbs and Spices

- Ginger, turmeric, garlic, parsley
- Add flavor without salt
- Some may reduce liver inflammation

Harmful Foods: What to Avoid and Why

Some foods make your liver work harder. They worsen inflammation. They raise fluid retention. They speed up damage. If you have cirrhosis, avoid these completely or limit them strictly.

High-Sodium Foods

- Canned soups, frozen dinners, processed meats, chips
- Cause water retention and swelling
- Increase pressure in the liver's blood vessels
- Aim for less than 2,000 mg sodium per day

Fried and Fatty Foods

- Fast food, bacon, sausage, butter, creamy sauces
- High in saturated fat
- Overload the liver's ability to process fa
- Can lead to fatty liver on top of cirrhosis

Sugary Foods and Drinks

- Candy, soda, pastries, sweetened yogurt
- Contribute to fat buildup in the liver
- Spike blood sugar and insulin levels
- Replace with fruit or low-sugar alternatives

Red Meat

- Beef, pork, lamb
- Harder to digest
- High in saturated fat and iron, which can stress the liver
- Replace with fish or poultry

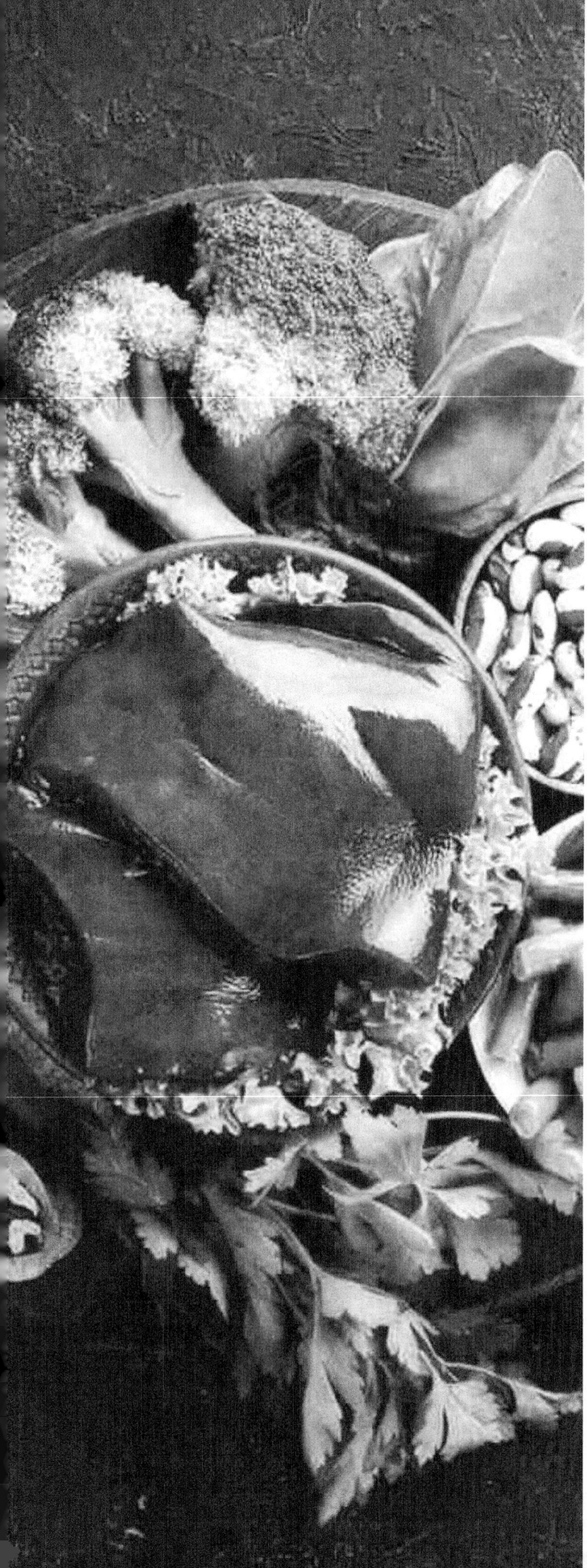

Herbal Supplements Without Approval

- Some herbs like comfrey, kava, and chaparral harm the liver
- Always check with your doctor before taking any supplement

Alcohol

- Beer, wine, liquor in any amount
- Directly damages liver cells
- Speeds up cirrhosis progression
- Must be completely avoided

Raw or Undercooked Shellfish

- Oysters, clams, mussels
- Risk of bacteria that a damaged liver cannot fight
- Cook all seafood thoroughly

Your liver is already working at a disadvantage. The wrong foods push it further. Stick to what helps. Avoid what hurts. Every meal is a chance to protect what remains.

CHAPTER 03

ESSENTIAL INGREDIENTS & KITCHEN TIPS

Shopping List for a Liver-Friendly Diet

Eating well starts with what you bring home. A liver-friendly kitchen begins at the store. This list helps you shop with purpose. It focuses on whole foods that support your liver and reduce stress on your body. Each item fits within the guidelines for cirrhosis—low sodium, low fat, high nutrition. Use this list to plan meals, fill your pantry, and keep cooking simple

Produce

- Broccoli
- Spinach
- Kale
- Carrots
- Beets
- Sweet potatoes
- Zucchini
- Bell peppers
- Cucumbers
- Tomatoes
- Onions
- Garlic
- Apples
- Berries (blueberries, strawberries)
- Bananas
- Oranges
- Grapes
- Lemons

Grains & Starches

- Brown rice
- Quinoa
- Oats (plain, unsweetened)
- Whole wheat pasta
- Barley
- Whole grain bread (low-sodium)

Protein

- Skinless chicken breast
- Turkey breast
- White fish (cod, tilapia)
- Salmon (in moderation)
- Eggs
- Tofu
- Tempeh
- Lentils
- Chickpeas
- Black beans
- Low-sodium canned beans (rinse before use)

Dairy & Alternatives

- Low-fat milk
- Plain Greek yogurt
- Cottage cheese
- Unsweetened almond or oat milk

Healthy Fats

- Olive oil
- Avocados
- Flaxseeds
- Chia seeds
- Walnuts

Herbs & Spices

- Fresh parsley
- Basil
- Oregano
- Ginger
- Turmeric
- Black pepper
- Cumin
- Cinnamon

Beverages

- Water
- Herbal teas (approved by doctor)
- Coconut water (low in sugar)

Pantry Staples

- Low-sodium vegetable broth
- No-salt-added canned tomatoes
- Natural peanut or almond butter (no added sugar or salt)
- Whole grain crackers (low-sodium)
- Apple cider vinegar

Essential Kitchen Equipment and Cooking Techniques

The right tools make healthy cooking easier. They save time. They reduce effort. They help you stick to your plan.

Recommended Equipment

- **Non-stick pans** – Cook with less oil
- **Steamer basket** – Preserve nutrients in vegetables
- **Blender** – Make smoothies and soups
- **Slow cooker** – Prep meals with less energy
- **Measuring cups/spoons** – Control portions and sodium
- **Digital food scale** – Track protein and portion sizes
- **Cutting board and sharp knives** – Speed up prep
- **Small saucepan** – Make single servings
- **Glass storage containers** – Store leftovers safely
- **Microwave-safe dishes** – Reheat meals with ease

Helpful Techniques

- **Steaming** – Keeps veggies tender without added fat
- **Baking** – Cooks evenly with no frying
- **Grilling** – Adds flavor without extra oil
- **Boiling or simmering** – Great for grains, legumes, and soups
- **Sautéing with broth** – Skip oil, keep flavor
- **Blending** – Use for purees, dressings, smoothies
- **Batch cooking** – Save energy and reduce decision fatigue

Keep meals simple. Avoid frying. Watch sauces and seasonings. Cook once, eat twice.

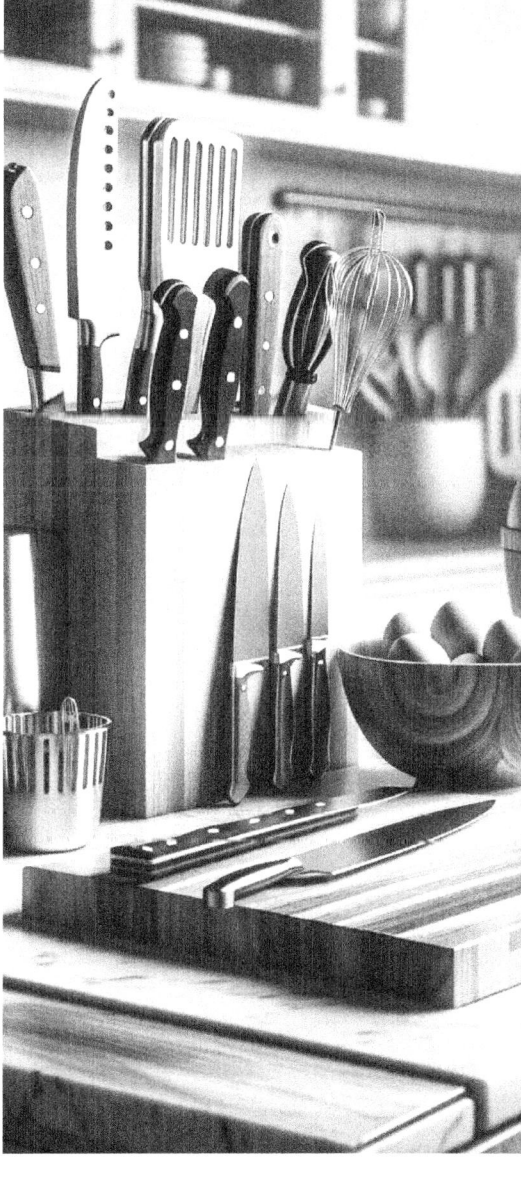

CHAPTER 04
BREAKFAST

Your first meal of the day is a prime opportunity to care for your liver. For seniors living with cirrhosis, breakfast is more than just calories; it's about creating a foundation of consistency, balance, and liver protection. The right breakfast supports stable blood sugar, healthy muscles, and comfortable digestion, while the wrong one can lead to unwelcome symptoms like bloating and fatigue.

Each meal prioritizes low-sodium, low-fat, high-protein ingredients and steers clear of processed foods, red meat, and anything that could burden your liver. Instead, these recipes focus on simple, nutrient-packed foods that are easy to digest and provide essential nourishment. Discover a range of appealing options, from comforting warm oats to energizing protein smoothies, versatile egg preparations, satisfying fiber toasts, and gentle porridges, with both plant-based and animal-protein choices.

These recipes are designed for quick preparation, requiring no complicated techniques or unusual ingredients. Make breakfast a simple and enjoyable part of your day. There's no need to skip it or resign yourself to bland choices. With the right guidance, breakfast can become a dependable tool for enhancing your strength, clarity, and overall well-being. These meals offer a straightforward and delicious way to start your day with intention and ease.

Berry Chia Pudding

- **Preparation Time:** 10 minutes
- **Cooking Time:** None (overnight refrigeration)
- **Servings:** 2

Ingredients:

- 1/4 cup chia seeds
- 1 cup unsweetened almond milk
- 1/2 cup fresh blueberries
- 1/2 cup fresh strawberries, sliced
- 1 tablespoon ground flaxseed
- 1 teaspoon honey (optional)

Instructions:

1. In a mixing bowl, combine chia seeds and almond milk. Stir well to prevent clumping.
2. Cover the bowl and refrigerate overnight to allow the mixture to thicken.
3. Before serving, stir the pudding to ensure even consistency.
4. Top with fresh blueberries, sliced strawberries, and a sprinkle of ground flaxseed.
5. Drizzle with honey if additional sweetness is desired.

Portion per Day:

- 1 serving (approximately 1 cup)

Nutritional Values (per serving):

- **Calories:** 180 kcal
- **Protein:** 5 g
- **Carbohydrates:** 20 g
- **Fats:** 9 g
- **Fiber:** 10 g
- **Sodium:** 50 mg
- **Cholesterol:** 0 mg

Oatmeal with Berries and Flaxseed

- **Preparation Time:** 5 minutes
- **Cooking Time:** 10 minutes
- **Servings:** 2

Ingredients:

- 1 cup rolled oats
- 2 cups water or unsweetened almond milk
- 1/2 cup fresh blueberries
- 1/2 cup sliced strawberries
- 1 tablespoon ground flaxseed
- 1 teaspoon honey (optional)

Instructions:

1. In a saucepan, bring water or almond milk to a boil.
2. Add rolled oats, reduce heat, and simmer for 5–7 minutes, stirring occasionally.
3. Once the oats are cooked, remove from heat and let sit for 2 minutes.
4. Divide the oatmeal into two bowls.
5. Top each serving with blueberries, strawberries, and a sprinkle of ground flaxseed.
6. Drizzle with honey if additional sweetness is desired.

Portion per Day: 1 serving (approximately 1 cup)

Nutritional Values (per serving):

- **Calories:** 220 kcal
- **Protein:** 6 g
- **Carbohydrates:** 38 g
- **Fats:** 5 g
- **Fiber:** 7 g
- **Sodium:** 50 mg
- **Cholesterol:** 0 mg

Greek Yogurt Parfait with Berries & Nuts

- **Preparation Time:** 5 minutes
- **Cooking Time:** None
- **Servings:** 1

Ingredients:

- 1 cup plain Greek yogurt (low-fat)
- 1/2 cup mixed berries (blueberries, raspberries, strawberries)
- 1 tablespoon chopped walnuts or almonds
- 1 teaspoon honey (optional)

Instructions:

1. In a serving glass or bowl, layer half of the Greek yogurt.
2. Add a layer of mixed berries.
3. Add the remaining yogurt on top.
4. Sprinkle with chopped nuts and drizzle with honey if desired.

Portion per Day: 1 serving

Nutritional Values (per serving):

- **Calories:** 250 kcal
- **Protein:** 20 g
- **Carbohydrates:** 15 g
- **Fats:** 12 g
- **Fiber:** 3 g
- **Sodium:** 70 mg
- **Cholesterol:** 10 mg

Quinoa Breakfast Bowl

- **Preparation Time:** 10 minutes
- **Cooking Time:** 15 minutes
- **Servings:** 2

Ingredients:

- 1 cup cooked quinoa
- 1/2 cup unsweetened almond milk
- 1/2 cup diced apples
- 1 tablespoon chopped walnuts
- 1/2 teaspoon cinnamon

Instructions:

1. In a saucepan, combine cooked quinoa and almond milk. Heat over medium heat until warm.
2. Stir in diced apples and cinnamon. Cook for 5 minutes.
3. Divide into bowls and top with chopped walnuts.

Portion per Day: 1 serving

Nutritional Values (per serving):

- **Calories:** 250 kcal
- **Protein:** 8 g
- **Carbohydrates:** 35 g
- **Fats:** 9 g
- **Fiber:** 5 g
- **Sodium:** 30 mg
- **Cholesterol:** 0 mg

Sweet Potato and Egg Hash

- **Preparation Time:** 10 minutes
- **Cooking Time:** 15 minutes
- **Servings:** 2

Ingredients:

- 1 medium sweet potato, diced
- 1/2 onion, chopped
- 1 tablespoon olive oil
- 2 eggs
- Fresh parsley for garnish

Instructions:

1. In a skillet, heat olive oil over medium heat. Add sweet potato and onion; cook until tender.
2. Create two wells in the hash and crack an egg into each. Cover and cook until eggs are set.
3. Garnish with fresh parsley.

Portion per Day: 1 serving

Nutritional Values (per serving):

- **Calories:** 300 kcal
- **Protein:** 10 g
- **Carbohydrates:** 30 g
- **Fats:** 15 g
- **Fiber:** 5 g
- **Sodium:** 70 mg
- **Cholesterol:** 185 mg

Spinach and Mushroom Omelette

- **Preparation Time:** 5 minutes
- **Cooking Time:** 10 minutes
- **Servings:** 1

Ingredients:

- 2 eggs
- 1/2 cup fresh spinach
- 1/4 cup sliced mushrooms
- 1 teaspoon olive oil

Instructions:

1. In a skillet, heat olive oil over medium heat. Sauté mushrooms until tender.
2. Add spinach and cook until wilted.
3. Beat eggs and pour over vegetables. Cook until set, then fold and serve.

Portion per Day: 1 serving

Nutritional Values (per serving):

- **Calories:** 200 kcal
- **Protein:** 14 g
- **Carbohydrates:** 3 g
- **Fats:** 15 g
- **Fiber:** 1 g
- **Sodium:** 140 mg
- **Cholesterol:** 370 mg

Banana Oat Pancakes

- **Preparation Time:** 10 minutes
- **Cooking Time:** 10 minutes
- **Servings:** 2

Ingredients:

- 1 ripe banana
- 1/2 cup rolled oats
- 2 eggs
- 1/2 teaspoon baking powder
- 1/2 teaspoon cinnamon

Instructions:

1. In a blender, combine all ingredients until smooth.
2. Heat a non-stick skillet over medium heat. Pour batter to form pancakes.
3. Cook until bubbles form, flip, and cook until golden brown.

Portion per Day: 1 serving

Nutritional Values (per serving):

- **Calories:** 250 kcal
- **Protein:** 10 g
- **Carbohydrates:** 30 g
- **Fats:** 10 g
- **Fiber:** 4 g
- **Sodium:** 150 mg
- **Cholesterol:** 185 mg

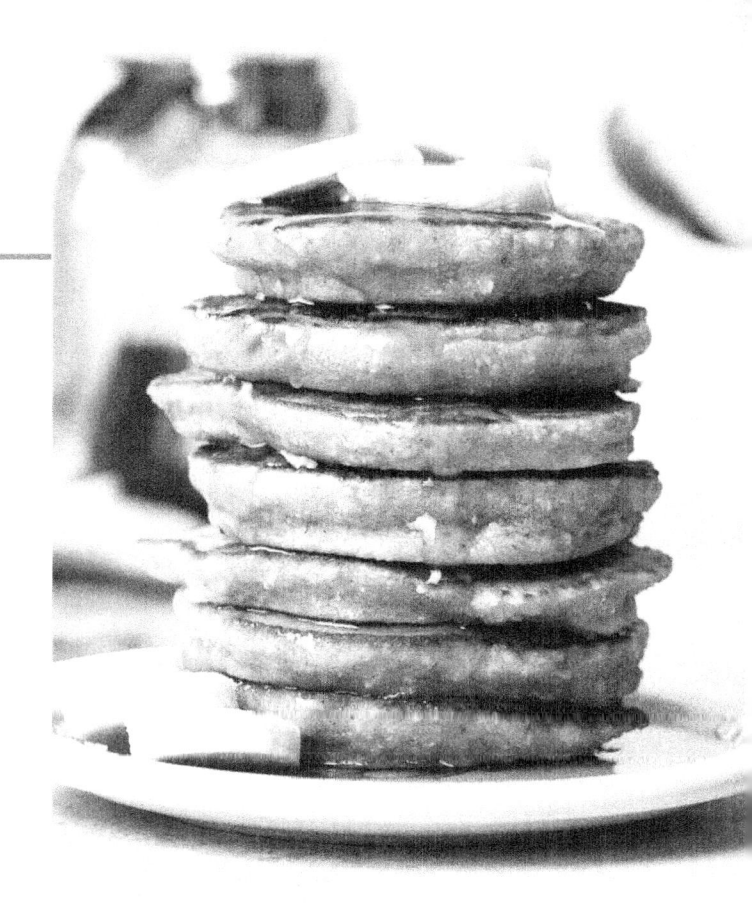

Cottage Cheese with Pineapple

- **Preparation Time:** 5 minutes
- **Cooking Time:** None
- **Servings:** 1

Ingredients:

- 1/2 cup low-fat cottage cheese
- 1/2 cup fresh pineapple chunks

Instructions:

1. In a bowl, combine cottage cheese and pineapple chunks.
2. Serve immediately.

Portion per Day: 1 serving

Nutritional Values (per serving):

- **Calories:** 150 kcal
- **Protein:** 14 g
- **Carbohydrates:** 12 g
- **Fats:** 5 g
- **Fiber:** 1 g
- **Sodium:** 400 mg
- **Cholesterol:** 20 mg

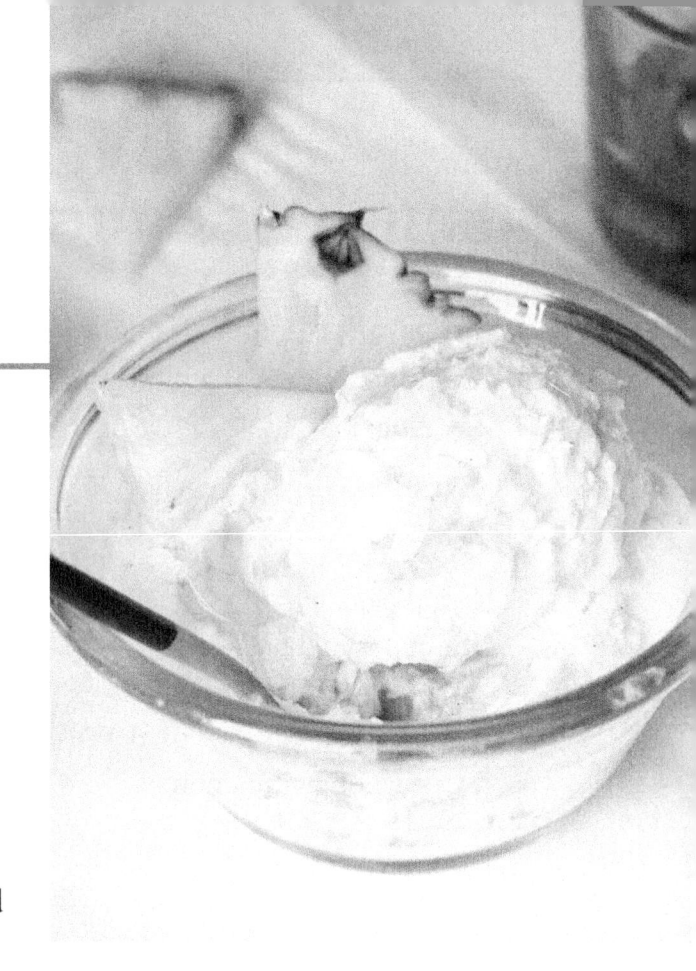

Vegetable Breakfast Wrap

- **Preparation Time:** 10 minutes
- **Cooking Time:** 5 minutes
- **Servings:** 1

Ingredients:

- 1 whole-grain tortilla
- 2 egg whites
- 1/4 cup chopped spinach
- 1/4 cup diced tomatoes
- 1/4 cup diced bell peppers
- 1 tablespoon low-fat shredded cheese (optional)

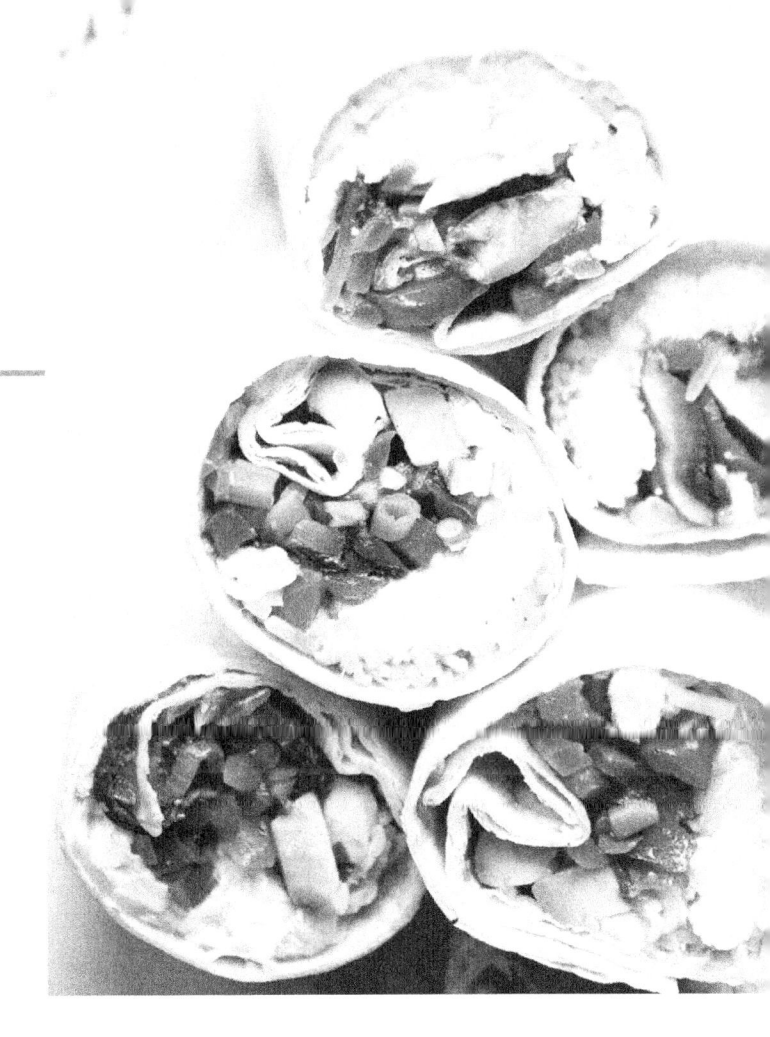

Instructions:

1. In a non-stick skillet, cook egg whites over medium heat until set.
2. Add spinach, tomatoes, and bell peppers; cook for 2–3 minutes.
3. Place the mixture onto the tortilla, sprinkle with cheese if using, and wrap.

Portion per Day: 1 wrap

Nutritional Values (per serving):

- **Calories:** 200 kcal
- **Protein:** 15 g
- **Carbohydrates:** 20 g
- **Fats:** 5 g
- **Fiber:** 4 g
- **Sodium:** 150 mg
- **Cholesterol:** 0 mg

Apple Cinnamon Quinoa

- **Preparation Time:** 5 minutes
- **Cooking Time:** 15 minutes
- **Servings:** 2

Ingredients:

- 1/2 cup quinoa
- 1 cup water
- 1 apple, diced
- 1/2 teaspoon cinnamon
- 1 teaspoon honey (optional)

Instructions:

1. Rinse quinoa and combine with water in a saucepan; bring to a boil.
2. Reduce heat, add diced apple and cinnamon, and simmer for 15 minutes.
3. Drizzle with honey before serving if desired.

Portion per Day: 1 serving

Nutritional Values (per serving):

- **Calories:** 220 kcal
- **Protein:** 6 g
- **Carbohydrates:** 40 g
- **Fats:** 3 g
- **Fiber:** 5 g
- **Sodium:** 10 mg
- **Cholesterol:** 0 mg

Avocado and Tomato Toast

- **Preparation Time:** 5 minutes
- **Cooking Time:** 5 minutes
- **Servings:** 1

Ingredients:

- 1 slice whole-grain bread
- 1/2 avocado, mashed
- 2 slices tomato
- 1 teaspoon lemon juice
- Freshly ground black pepper to taste

Instructions:

1. Toast the bread slice.
2. Spread mashed avocado mixed with lemon juice onto the toast.
3. Top with tomato slices and sprinkle with black pepper.

Portion per Day: 1 slice

Nutritional Values (per serving):

- **Calories:** 250 kcal
- **Protein:** 5 g
- **Carbohydrates:** 20 g
- **Fats:** 18 g
- **Fiber:** 7 g
- **Sodium:** 150 mg
- **Cholesterol:** 0 mg

Berry Smoothie Bowl

- **Preparation Time:** 5 minutes
- **Cooking Time:** None
- **Servings:** 1

Ingredients:

- 1/2 cup unsweetened almond milk
- 1/2 cup mixed berries (blueberries, raspberries, strawberries)
- 1/2 banana
- 1 tablespoon chia seeds
- 1 tablespoon sliced almonds

Instructions:

1. Blend almond milk, berries, banana, and chia seeds until smooth.
2. Pour into a bowl and top with sliced almonds.

Portion per Day: 1 bowl

Nutritional Values (per serving):

- **Calories:** 200 kcal
- **Protein:** 4 g
- **Carbohydrates:** 30 g
- **Fats:** 8 g
- **Fiber:** 6 g
- **Sodium:** 50 mg
- **Cholesterol:** 0 mg

Tofu Scramble

- **Preparation Time:** 10 minutes
- **Cooking Time:** 10 minutes
- **Servings:** 2

Ingredients:

- 1/2 block firm tofu, crumbled
- 1/4 cup diced bell peppers
- 1/4 cup chopped spinach
- 1/4 teaspoon turmeric
- 1 tablespoon olive oil

Instructions:

1. Heat olive oil in a skillet over medium heat.
2. Add bell peppers and cook for 2 minutes.
3. Add crumbled tofu, spinach, and turmeric; cook for 5–7 minutes.

Portion per Day: 1 serving

Nutritional Values (per serving):

- **Calories:** 180 kcal
- **Protein:** 12 g
- **Carbohydrates:** 5 g
- **Fats:** 12 g
- **Fiber:** 2 g
- **Sodium:** 150 mg
- **Cholesterol:** 0 mg

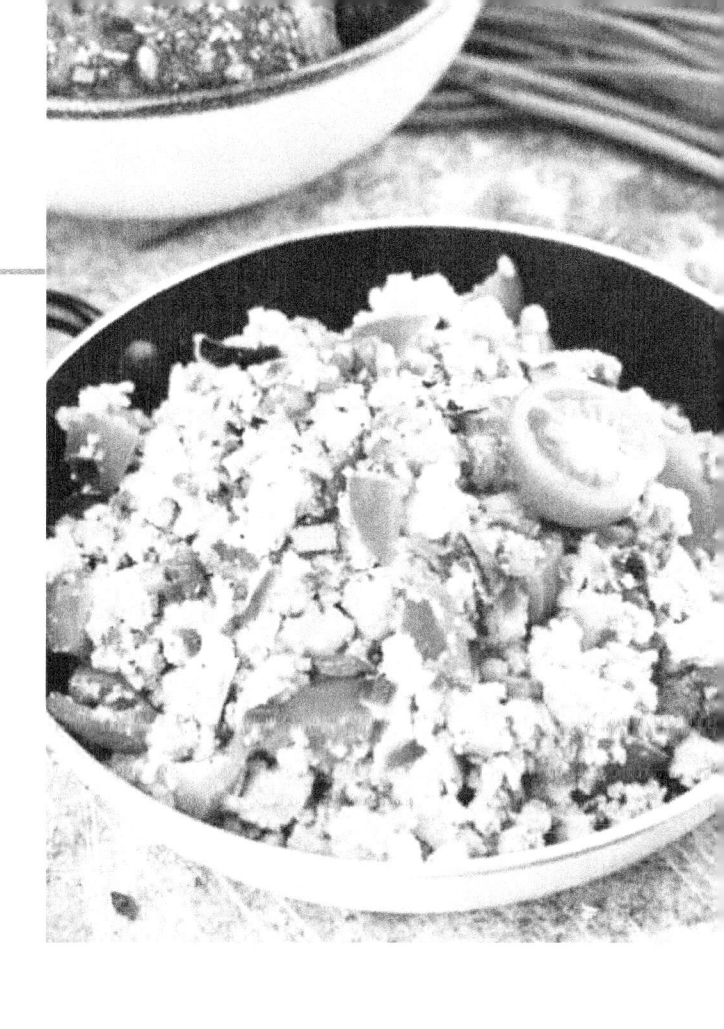

Sweet Potato and Black Bean Hash

- **Preparation Time:** 10 minutes
- **Cooking Time:** 15 minutes
- **Servings:** 2

Ingredients:

- 1 medium sweet potato, diced
- 1/2 cup cooked black beans
- 1/4 cup diced red bell pepper
- 1 tablespoon olive oil
- 1/4 teaspoon cumin

Instructions:

1. Heat olive oil in a skillet over medium heat.
2. Add sweet potato and cook until tender.
3. Add black beans, bell pepper, and cumin; cook for 5 minutes.

Portion per Day: 1 serving

Nutritional Values (per serving):

- **Calories:** 250 kcal
- **Protein:** 8 g
- **Carbohydrates:** 35 g
- **Fats:** 8 g
- **Fiber:** 7 g
- **Sodium:** 150 mg
- **Cholesterol:** 0 mg

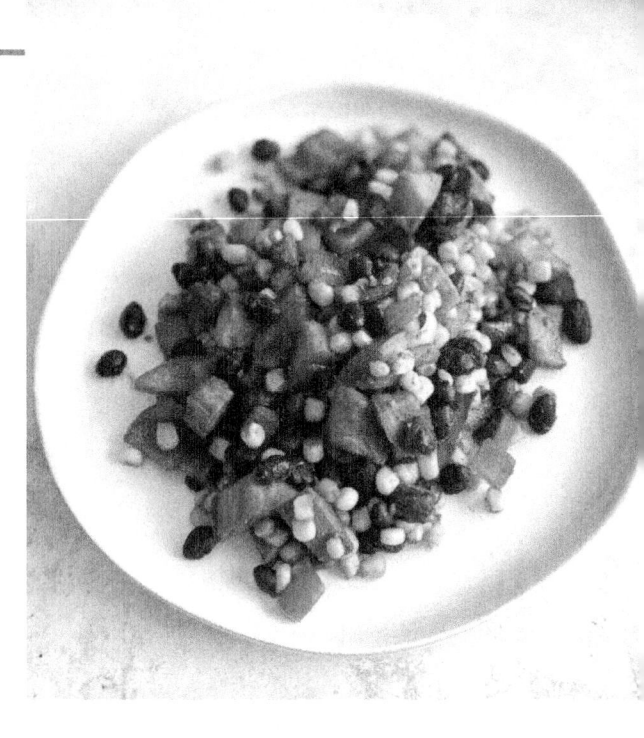

Greek Yogurt with Walnuts and Honey

- **Preparation Time:** 5 minutes
- **Cooking Time:** None
- **Servings:** 1

Ingredients:

- 1 cup plain Greek yogurt (low-fat)
- 1 tablespoon chopped walnuts
- 1 teaspoon honey

Instructions:

1. In a bowl, combine Greek yogurt, walnuts, and honey.
2. Serve immediately.

Portion per Day: 1 serving

Nutritional Values (per serving):

- **Calories:** 200 kcal
- **Protein:** 18 g
- **Carbohydrates:** 10 g
- **Fats:** 10 g
- **Fiber:** 1 g
- **Sodium:** 70 mg
- **Cholesterol:** 10 mg

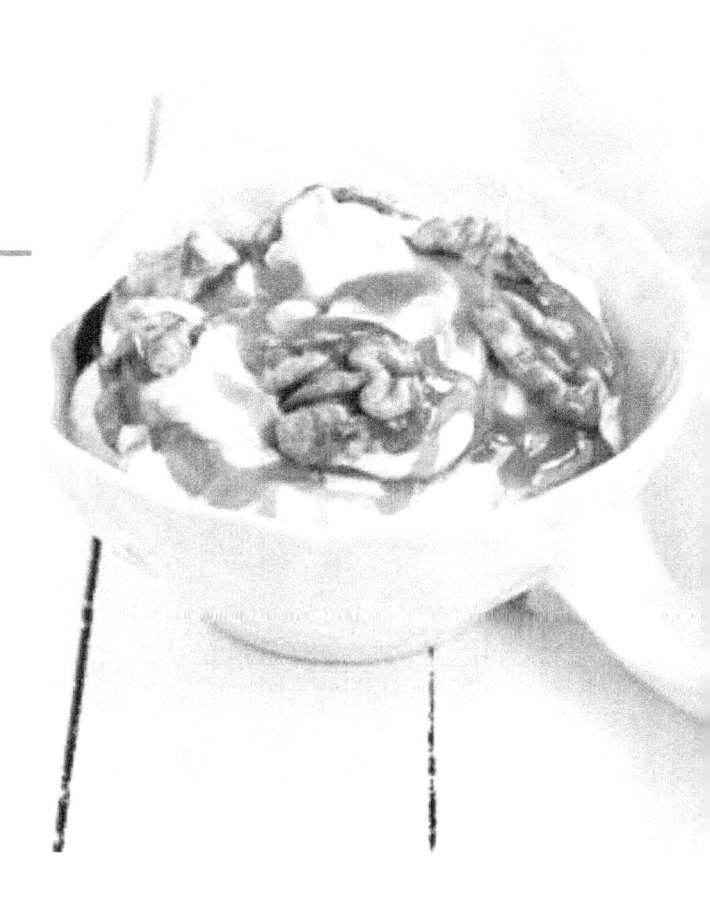

Whole Grain Toast with Almond Butter and Banana

- **Preparation Time:** 5 minutes
- **Cooking Time:** 2 minutes
- **Servings:** 1

Ingredients:

- 1 slice whole-grain bread
- 1 tablespoon almond butter
- 1/2 banana, sliced

Instructions:

1. Toast the bread slice.
2. Spread almond butter over the toast.
3. Top with banana slices.

Portion per Day: 1 slice

Nutritional Values (per serving):

- **Calories:** 250 kcal
- **Protein:** 6 g
- **Carbohydrates:** 30 g
- **Fats:** 12 g
- **Fiber:** 5 g
- **Sodium:** 150 mg
- **Cholesterol:** 0 mg

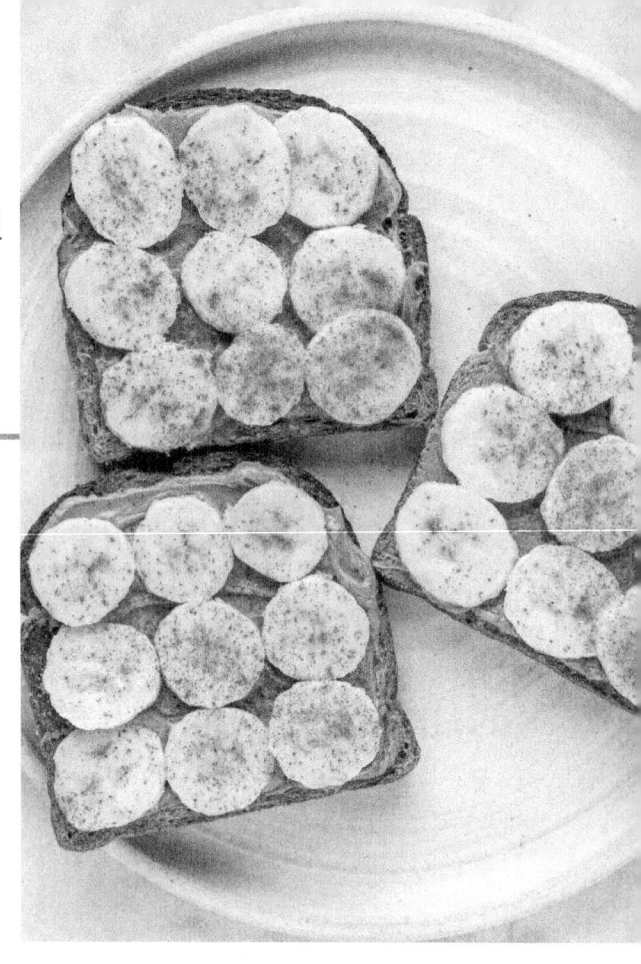

Vegetable and Tofu Stir-Fry

- **Preparation Time:** 10 minutes
- **Cooking Time:** 10 minutes
- **Servings:** 2

Ingredients:

- 1/2 block firm tofu, cubed
- 1/2 cup broccoli florets
- 1/2 cup sliced bell peppers
- 1 tablespoon olive oil
- 1 teaspoon low-sodium soy sauce

Instructions:

1. Heat olive oil in a skillet over medium heat.
2. Add tofu cubes and cook until golden brown.
3. Add broccoli and bell peppers; stir-fry for 5 minutes.
4. Drizzle with low-sodium soy sauce before serving.

Portion per Day: 1 serving

Nutritional Values (per serving):

- **Calories:** 220 kcal
- **Protein:** 14 g
- **Carbohydrates:** 10 g
- **Fats:** 14 g
- **Fiber:** 4 g
- **Sodium:** 200 mg
- **Cholesterol:** 0 mg

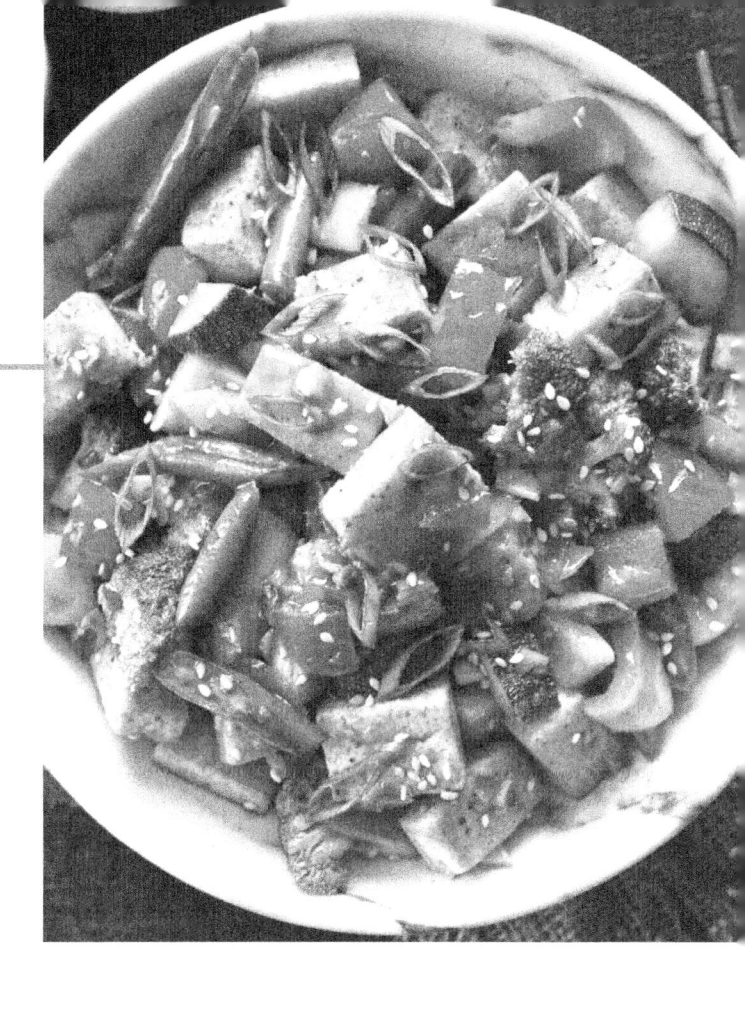

Oatmeal with Sliced Apples and Cinnamon

- **Preparation Time:** 5 minutes
- **Cooking Time:** 10 minutes
- **Servings:** 2

Ingredients:

- 1 cup rolled oats
- 2 cups water or unsweetened almond milk
- 1 apple, thinly sliced
- 1/2 teaspoon cinnamon

Instructions:

1. In a saucepan, bring water or almond milk to a boil.
2. Add oats and cook for 5 minutes.
3. Stir in apple slices and cinnamon; cook for an additional 5 minutes.

Portion per Day: 1 serving

Nutritional Values (per serving):

- **Calories:** 200 kcal
- **Protein:** 5 g
- **Carbohydrates:** 35 g
- **Fats:** 4 g
- **Fiber:** 6 g
- **Sodium:** 50 mg
- **Cholesterol:** 0 mg

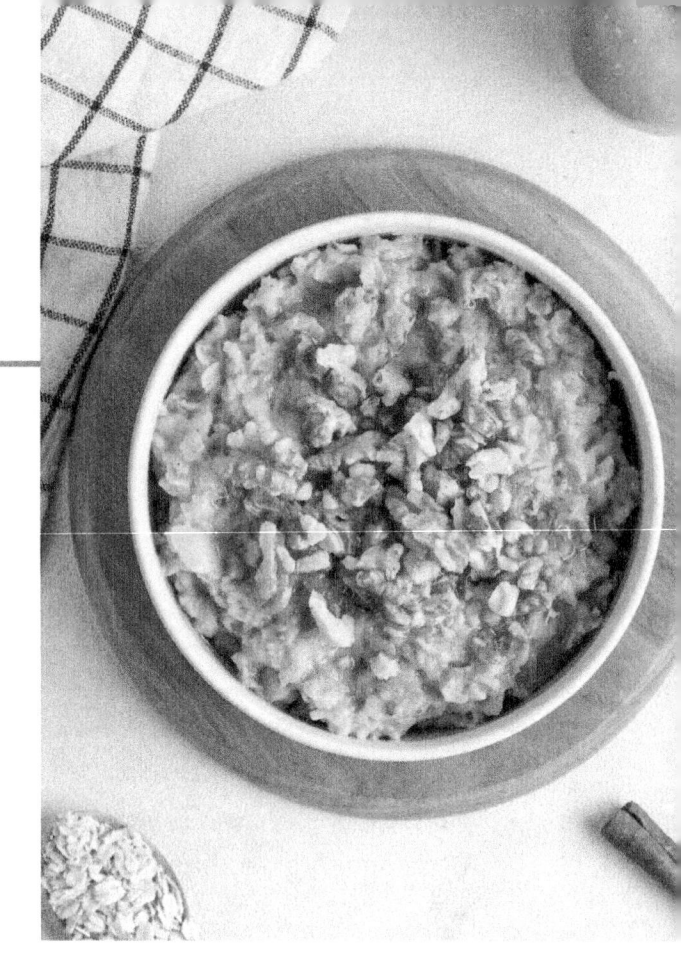

Smoothie with Spinach, Banana, and Flaxseed

- **Preparation Time:** 5 minutes
- **Cooking Time:** None
- **Servings:** 1

Ingredients:

- 1 cup unsweetened almond milk
- 1/2 banana
- 1 cup fresh spinach
- 1 tablespoon ground flaxseed

Instructions:

1. Combine all ingredients in a blender.
2. Blend until smooth and serve immediately.

Portion per Day: 1 serving

Nutritional Values (per serving):

- **Calories:** 180 kcal
- **Protein:** 4 g
- **Carbohydrates:** 20 g
- **Fats:** 8 g
- **Fiber:** 5 g
- **Sodium:** 60 mg
- **Cholesterol:** 0 mg

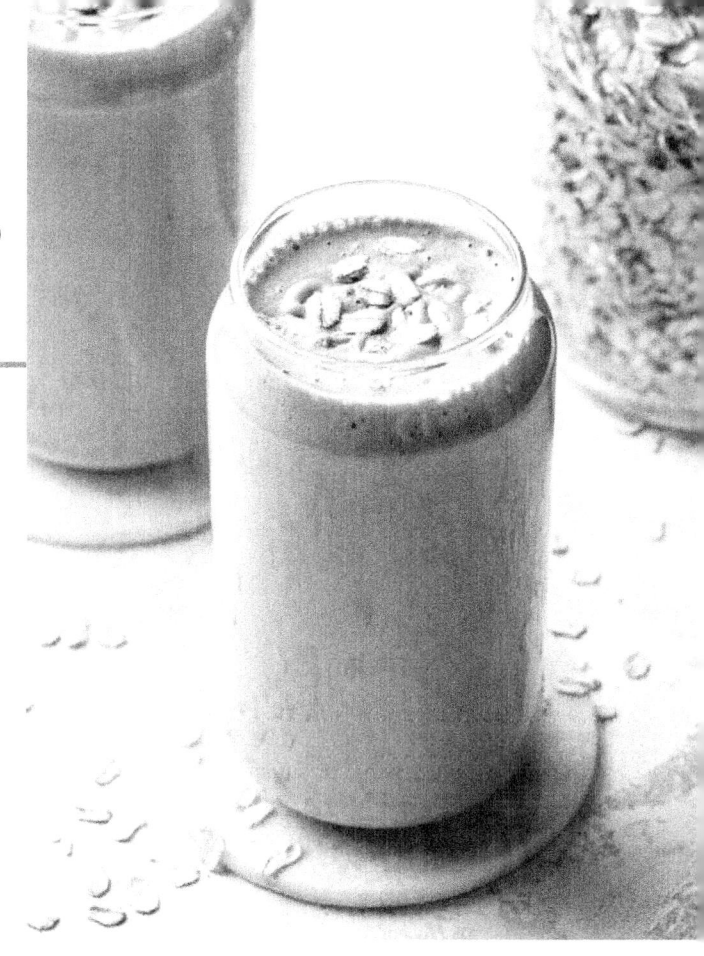

Cottage Cheese & Berry Wrap

- **Preparation Time:** 10 minutes
- **Cooking Time:** None
- **Servings:** 2

Ingredients:

- 1 cup low-fat cottage cheese
- ½ cup blueberries
- ½ cup strawberries, sliced
- 2 whole grain wraps
- 1 tbsp ground flaxseed

Instructions:

1. Spread cottage cheese on wraps.
2. Top with berries and flaxseed.
3. Roll and slice for easy eating.

Portion per Day: 1 wrap

Nutritional Values (per serving):

- **Calories:** 290
- **Protein:** 21g
- **Carbohydrates:** 28g
- **Fats:** 9g
- **Fiber:** 6g
- **Sodium:** 105mg
- **Cholesterol:** 15mg

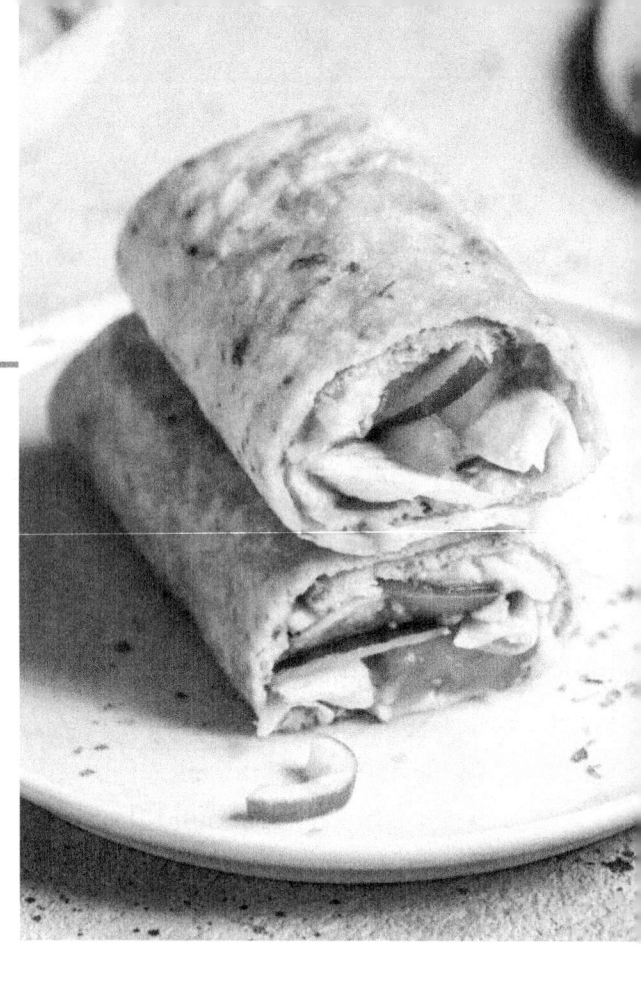

Egg White and Veggie Scramble with Toast

- **Preparation Time:** 10 minutes
- **Cooking Time:** 10 minutes
- **Servings:** 2

Ingredients:

- 4 egg whites
- 1 cup spinach
- ½ bell pepper, chopped
- 1 tsp olive oil
- 2 slices whole grain low-sodium bread

Instructions:

1. Sauté veggies in olive oil for 3 minutes.
2. Add egg whites and cook while stirring until set.
3. Serve with toasted bread.

Portion per Day: 1 egg scramble and 1 slice toast

Nutritional Values (per serving):

- **Calories:** 220
- **Protein:** 19g
- **Carbohydrates**: 17g
- **Fats:** 6g
- **Fiber:** 4g
- **Sodium:** 100mg
- **Cholesterol:** 0mg

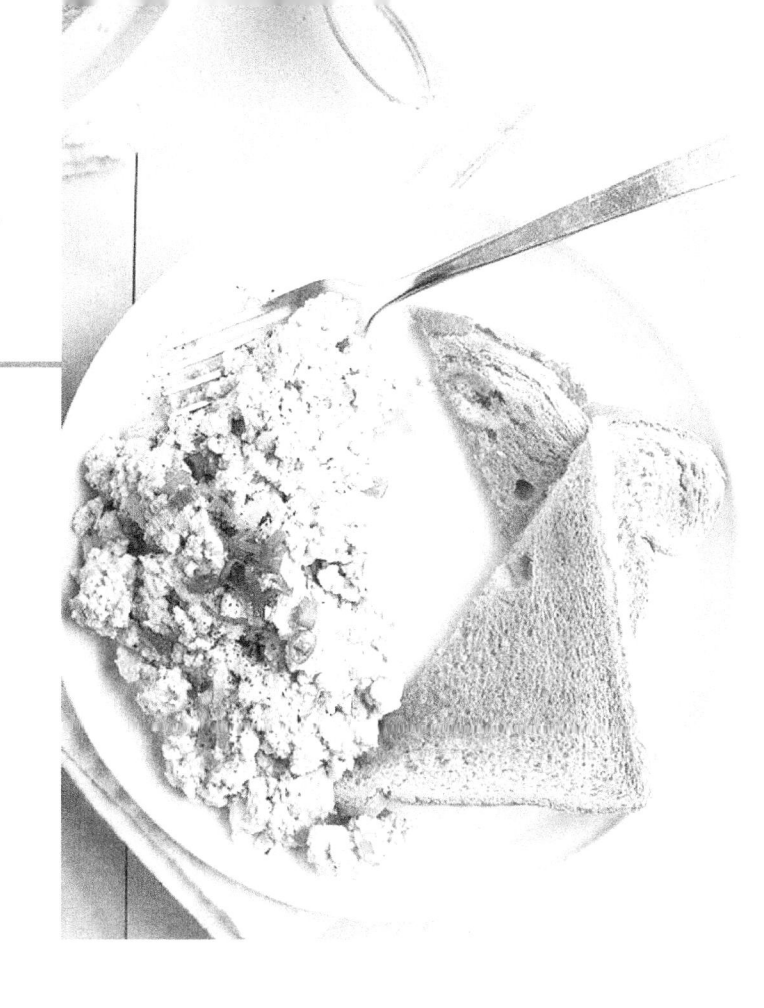

CHAPTER 05
LUNCHES

Lunch bridges the gap between morning energy and afternoon fatigue, making it crucial for seniors with liver cirrhosis. This midday meal must balance specific nutritional needs: sufficient protein for strength, adequate fiber for digestion, and liver-friendly nutrients—all while limiting sodium to manage fluid retention and blood pressure.

Finding satisfying lunches that meet these requirements can be challenging. The recipes in this collection solve this dilemma by featuring lean proteins, legumes, whole grains, and beneficial fats instead of liver-taxing fried foods, processed meats, or high-sodium options.

Designed with simplicity in mind, these high-protein, low-sodium meals—including wraps, salads, soups, bowls, and stir-fries—use accessible ingredients and straightforward preparation methods. They provide the variety and structure you need while supporting your health, leaving you nourished and comfortable after eating.

Quinoa and Black Bean Bowl

- **Preparation Time:** 10 minutes
- **Cooking Time:** 15 minutes
- **Servings:** 2

Ingredients:

- 1 cup cooked quinoa
- 1 cup canned black beans (no salt added), rinsed
- 1/2 red bell pepper, diced
- 1/4 cup chopped fresh cilantro
- Juice of 1 lime
- 1 tablespoon olive oil

Instructions:

1. In a bowl, combine quinoa, black beans, bell pepper, and cilantro.
2. Drizzle with lime juice and olive oil; toss to combine.

Portion per Day: 1 serving

Nutritional Values (per serving):

- **Calories:** 310 kcal
- **Protein:** 14 g
- **Carbohydrates:** 40 g
- **Fats:** 10 g
- **Fiber:** 9 g
- **Sodium:** 100 mg
- **Cholesterol:** 0 mg

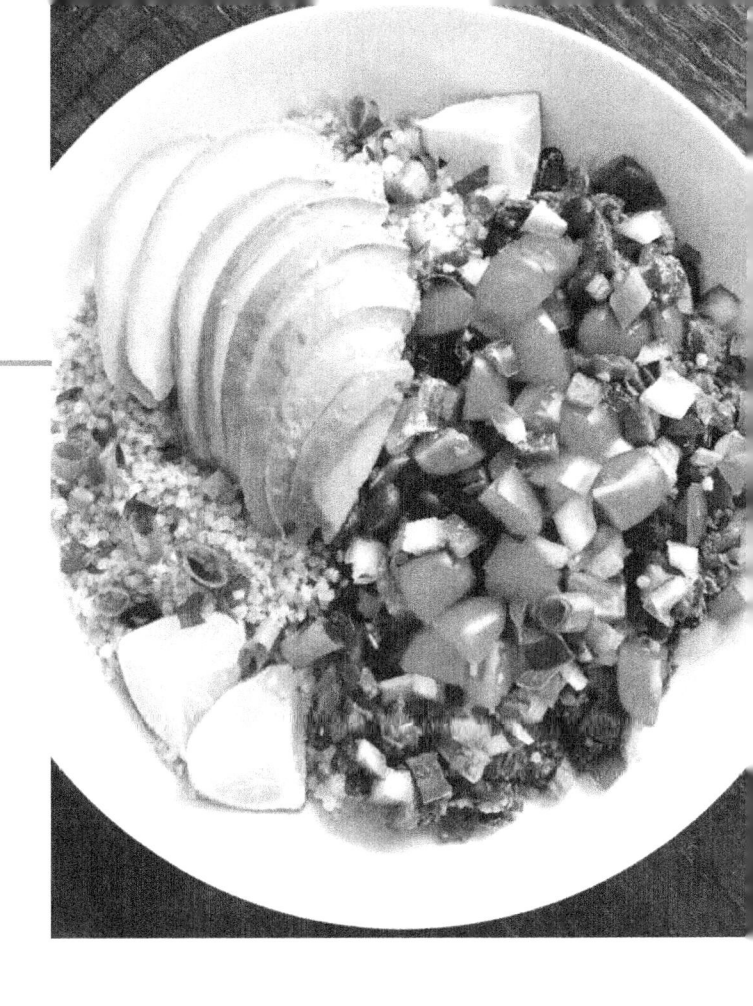

Turkey and Avocado Wrap

- **Preparation Time:** 10 minutes
- **Cooking Time:** None
- **Servings:** 1

Ingredients:

- 1 whole-grain tortilla
- 3 ounces sliced low-sodium turkey breast
- 1/2 avocado, sliced
- 1/2 cup shredded lettuce
- 1 small tomato, sliced

Instructions:

1. Lay tortilla flat and layer with turkey, avocado, lettuce, and tomato.
2. Roll up tightly and slice in half.

Portion per Day: 1 wrap

Nutritional Values (per serving):

- **Calories:** 350 kcal
- **Protein:** 25 g
- **Carbohydrates:** 30 g
- **Fats:** 18 g
- **Fiber:** 7 g
- **Sodium:** 140 mg
- **Cholesterol:** 50 mg

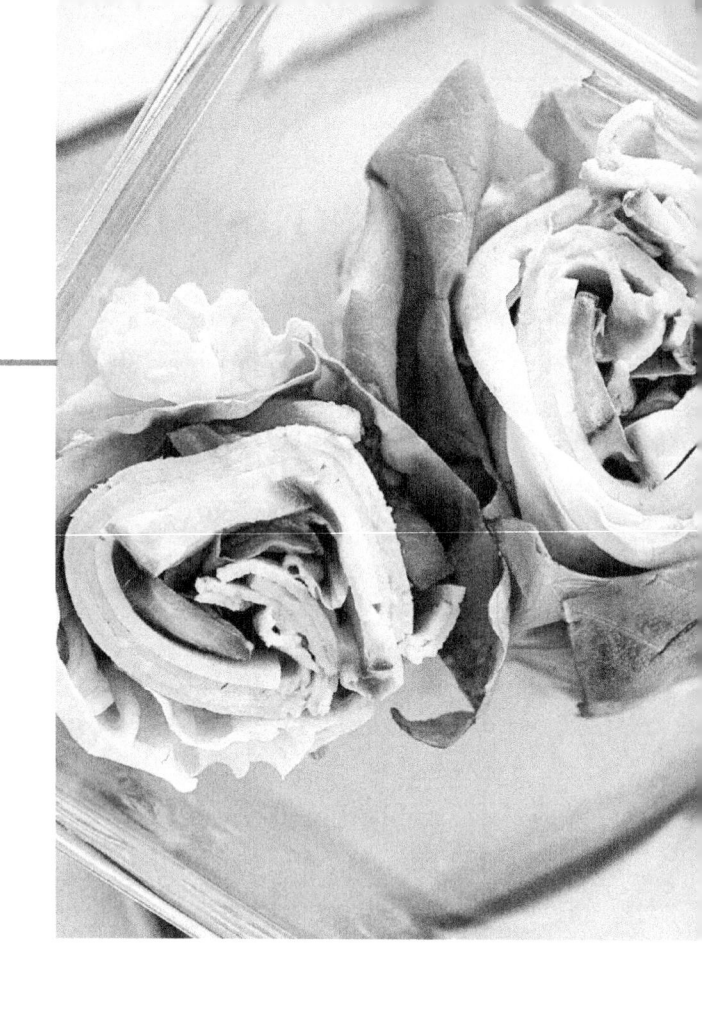

Lentil & Quinoa Salad

- **Preparation Time:** 10 minutes
- **Cooking Time:** 20 minutes
- **Servings:** 2

Ingredients:

- 1/2 cup cooked lentils
- 1/2 cup cooked quinoa
- 1/2 cup diced cucumber
- 1/2 cup cherry tomatoes, halved
- 1 tablespoon olive oil
- Juice of 1 lemon
- 1 tablespoon chopped fresh mint

Instructions:

1. In a bowl, combine lentils, quinoa, cucumber, and tomatoes.
2. Drizzle with olive oil and lemon juice.
3. Sprinkle with fresh mint and toss gently.

Portion per Day: 1 serving

Nutritional Values (per serving):

- **Calories:** 290 kcal
- **Protein:** 14 g
- **Carbohydrates:** 35 g
- **Fats:** 12 g
- **Fiber:** 9 g
- **Sodium:** 80 mg
- **Cholesterol:** 0 mg

Grilled Shrimp and Quinoa Bowl

- **Preparation Time:** 15 minutes
- **Cooking Time:** 10 minutes
- **Servings:** 2

Ingredients:

- 8 oz shrimp, peeled and deveined
- 1 cup cooked quinoa
- 1 cup steamed broccoli florets
- 1 tablespoon olive oil
- Juice of 1 lemon
- 1 teaspoon garlic powder

Instructions:

1. Toss shrimp with olive oil, lemon juice, and garlic powder.
2. Grill shrimp over medium heat until opaque.
3. In bowls, layer quinoa, broccoli, and grilled shrimp.

Portion per Day: 1 bowl

Nutritional Values (per serving):

- **Calories:** 320 kcal
- **Protein:** 28 g
- **Carbohydrates:** 30 g
- **Fats:** 10 g
- **Fiber:** 5 g
- **Sodium:** 120 mg
- **Cholesterol:** 180 mg

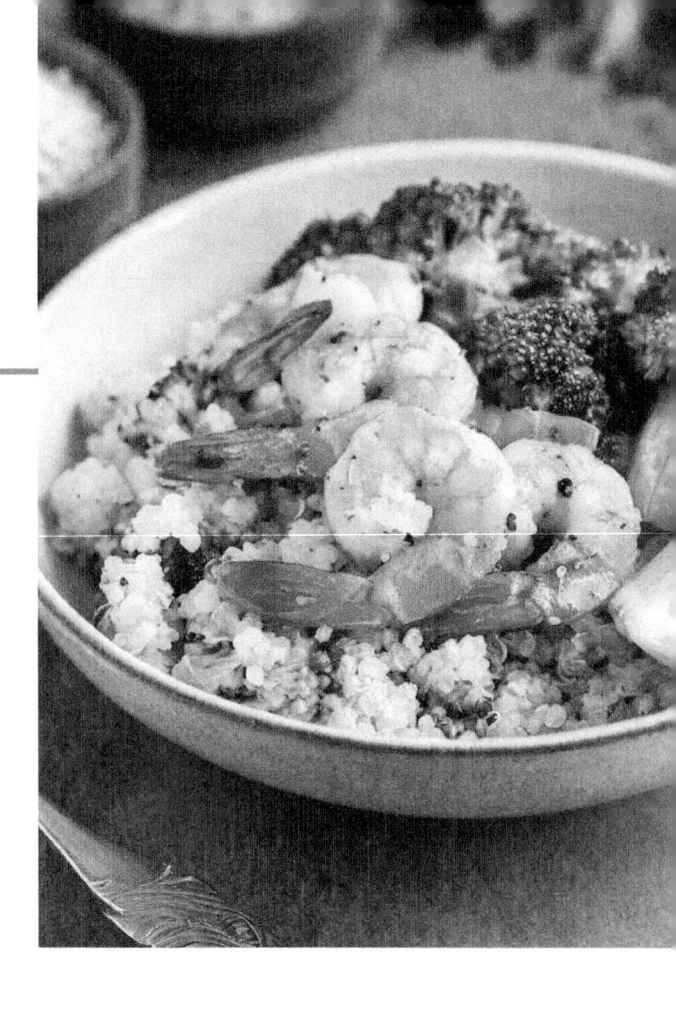

Lentil and Sweet Potato Stew

- **Preparation Time:** 10 minutes
- **Cooking Time:** 30 minutes
- **Servings:** 3

Ingredients:

- 1 cup dried lentils, rinsed
- 1 medium sweet potato, diced
- 1 small onion, chopped
- 2 cloves garlic, minced
- 4 cups low-sodium vegetable broth
- 1 teaspoon cumin

Instructions:

1. In a pot, sauté onion and garlic until translucent.
2. Add lentils, sweet potato, broth, and cumin.
3. Simmer for 30 minutes until lentils and sweet potato are tender.

Portion per Day: 1 serving

Nutritional Values (per serving):

- **Calories:** 310 kcal
- **Protein:** 16 g
- **Carbohydrates:** 45 g
- **Fats:** 5 g
- **Fiber:** 10 g
- **Sodium:** 100 mg
- **Cholesterol:** 0 mg

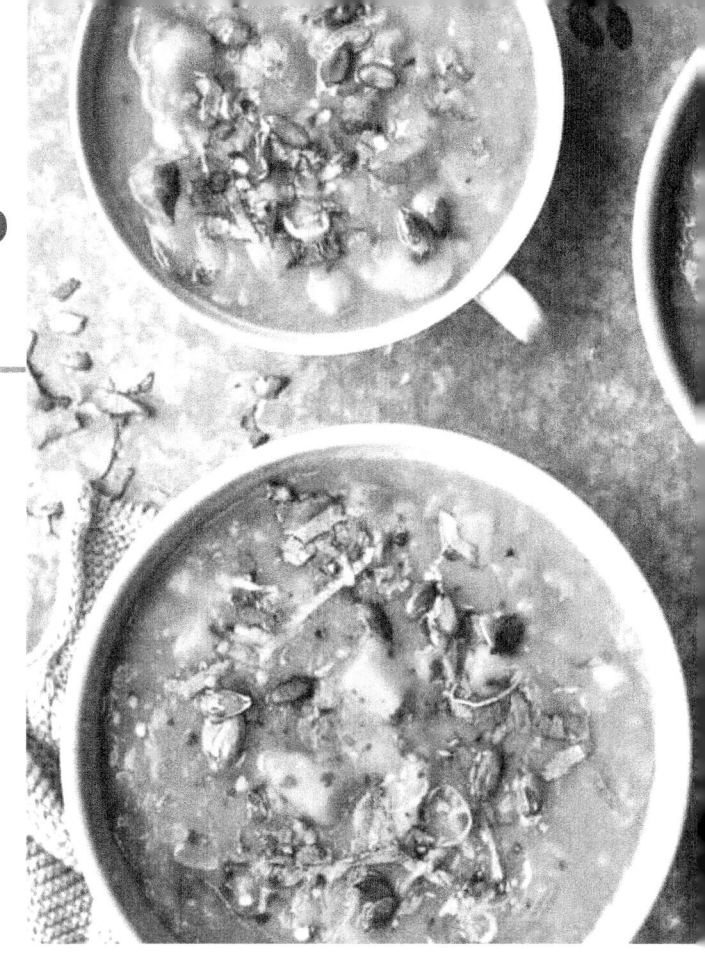

Grilled Turkey and Zucchini Skewers

- **Preparation Time:** 15 minutes
- **Cooking Time:** 10 minutes
- **Servings:** 2

Ingredients:

- 8 oz ground turkey (lean, no added salt)
- 1 zucchini, sliced
- 1 tablespoon fresh parsley, chopped
- 1 teaspoon garlic powder
- 1 tablespoon olive oil

Instructions:

1. In a bowl, mix ground turkey, parsley, and garlic powder.
2. Form small meatballs and thread onto skewers alternating with zucchini slices.
3. Brush with olive oil and grill until turkey is cooked through.

Portion per Day: 1 skewer

Nutritional Values (per serving):

- **Calories:** 280 kcal
- **Protein:** 30 g
- **Carbohydrates:** 5 g
- **Fats:** 16 g
- **Fiber:** 2 g
- **Sodium:** 95 mg
- **Cholesterol:** 75 mg

Eggplant and Chickpea Stir-Fry

- **Preparation Time:** 10 minutes
- **Cooking Time:** 15 minutes
- **Servings:** 2

Ingredients:

- 1 medium eggplant, diced
- 1 can (15 oz) no-salt-added chickpeas, drained and rinsed
- 1 tablespoon olive oil
- 1 teaspoon ground turmeric
- 1/2 teaspoon black pepper

Instructions:

1. In a skillet, heat olive oil over medium heat.
2. Add eggplant and cook until softened.
3. Stir in chickpeas, turmeric, and black pepper; cook for 5 more minutes.

Portion per Day: 1 serving

Nutritional Values (per serving):

- **Calories:** 270 kcal
- **Protein:** 10 g
- **Carbohydrates:** 30 g
- **Fats:** 12 g
- **Fiber:** 8 g
- **Sodium:** 85 mg
- **Cholesterol:** 0 mg

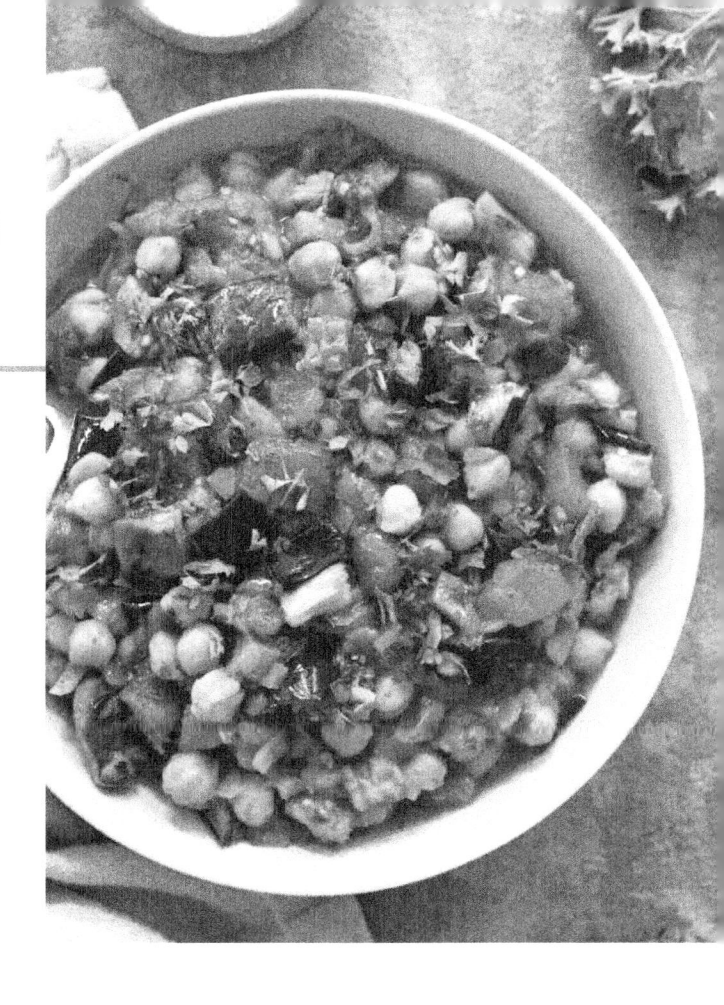

Baked Salmon with Dill Yogurt Sauce

- **Preparation Time:** 10 minutes
- **Cooking Time:** 15 minutes
- **Servings:** 2

Ingredients:

- 2 salmon fillets (4 oz each)
- 1 tablespoon olive oil
- 1/2 cup plain low-fat Greek yogurt
- 1 tablespoon fresh dill, chopped
- Juice of 1/2 lemon
- 1 garlic clove, minced

Instructions:

1. Preheat oven to 375°F (190°C).
2. Place salmon fillets on a baking sheet, drizzle with olive oil.
3. Bake for 15 minutes or until cooked through.
4. In a bowl, mix yogurt, dill, lemon juice, and garlic.
5. Serve salmon topped with dill yogurt sauce.

Portion per Day: 1 fillet

Nutritional Values (per serving):

- **Calories:** 320 kcal
- **Protein:** 35 g
- **Carbohydrates:** 4 g
- **Fats:** 18 g
- **Fiber:** 0 g
- **Sodium:** 85 mg
- **Cholesterol:** 70 mg

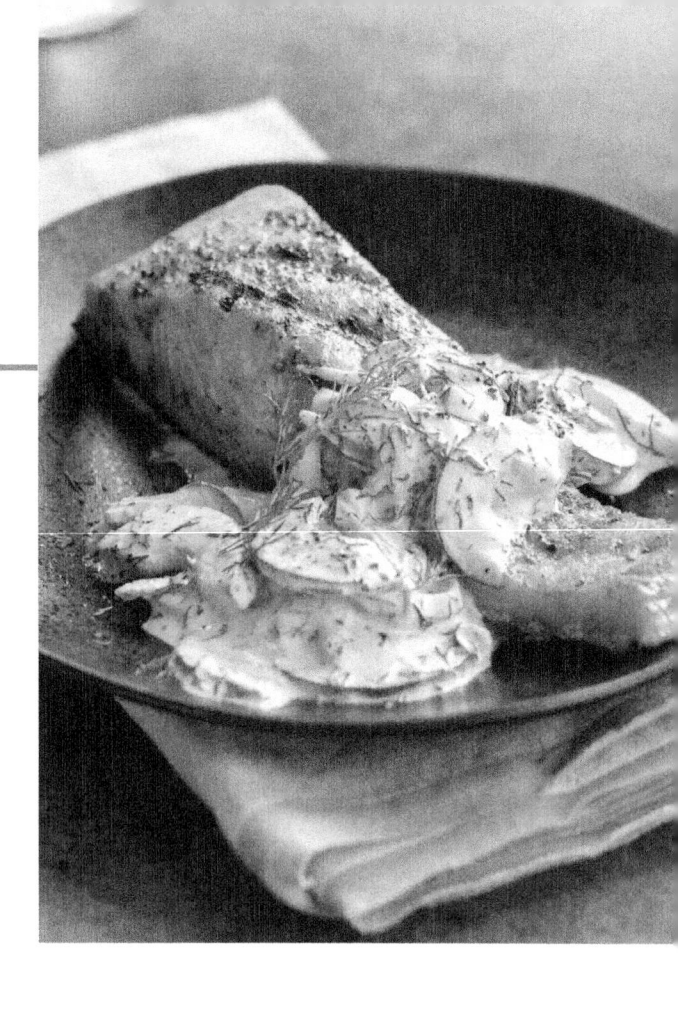

Chickpea and Spinach Stew

- **Preparation Time:** 10 minutes
- **Cooking Time:** 20 minutes
- **Servings:** 3

Ingredients:

- 1 can (15 oz) no-salt-added chickpeas, drained and rinsed
- 2 cups fresh spinach
- 1 small onion, diced
- 2 cloves garlic, minced
- 1 tablespoon olive oil
- 1 teaspoon ground cumin
- 2 cups low-sodium vegetable broth

Instructions:

1. In a pot, sauté onion and garlic in olive oil until translucent.
2. Add cumin, chickpeas, and broth; simmer for 15 minutes.
3. Stir in spinach and cook until wilted.

Portion per Day: 1 serving

Nutritional Values (per serving):

- **Calories:** 250 kcal
- **Protein:** 12 g
- **Carbohydrates:** 30 g
- **Fats:** 10 g
- **Fiber:** 8 g
- **Sodium:** 90 mg
- **Cholesterol:** 0 mg

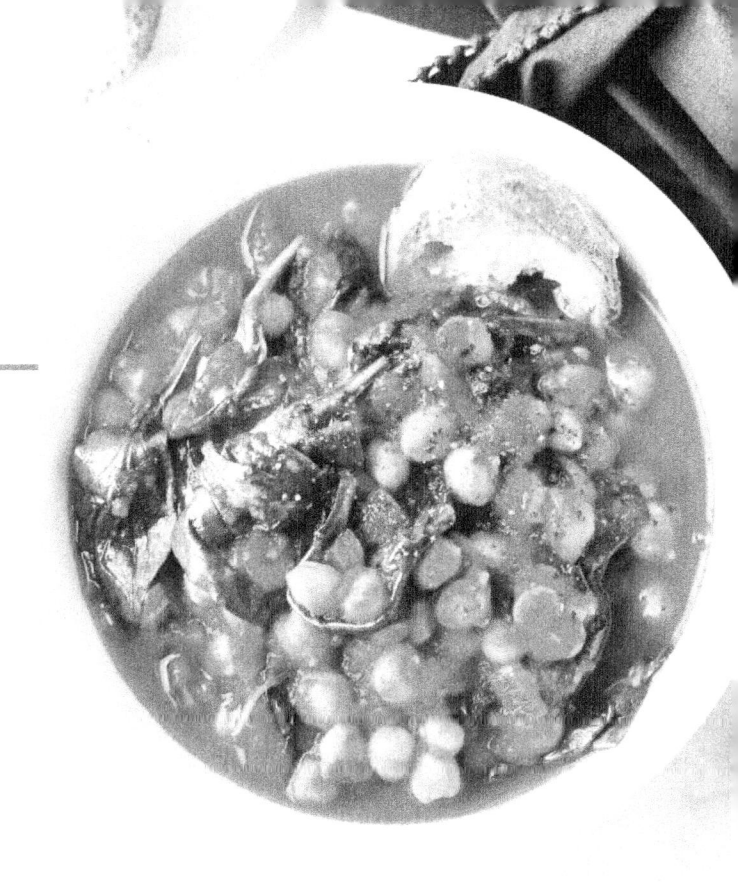

Lentil and Vegetable Soup

- **Preparation Time:** 15 minutes
- **Cooking Time:** 30 minutes
- **Servings:** 4

Ingredients:

- 1 cup dried lentils, rinsed
- 1 carrot, diced
- 1 celery stalk, diced
- 1 small onion, chopped
- 2 cloves garlic, minced
- 4 cups low-sodium vegetable broth
- 1 teaspoon dried thyme

Instructions:

1. In a large pot, sauté onion, carrot, celery, and garlic until softened.
2. Add lentils, broth, and thyme; bring to a boil.
3. Reduce heat and simmer for 30 minutes until lentils are tender.

Portion per Day: 1 serving

Nutritional Values (per serving):

- **Calories:** 220 kcal
- **Protein:** 15 g
- **Carbohydrates:** 35 g
- **Fats:** 3 g
- **Fiber:** 12 g
- **Sodium:** 90 mg
- **Cholesterol:** 0 mg

Grilled Tofu and Vegetable Skewers

- **Preparation Time:** 20 minutes
- **Cooking Time:** 10 minutes
- **Servings:** 2

Ingredients:

- 1 block firm tofu, cut into cubes
- 1 zucchini, sliced
- 1 red bell pepper, chopped
- 1 tablespoon olive oil
- 1 teaspoon dried basil

Instructions:

1. Toss tofu and vegetables with olive oil and basil.
2. Thread onto skewers and grill until browned.

Portion per Day: 1 serving

Nutritional Values (per serving):

- **Calories:** 300 kcal
- **Protein:** 20 g
- **Carbohydrates:** 10 g
- **Fats:** 20 g
- **Fiber:** 4 g
- **Sodium:** 80 mg
- **Cholesterol:** 0 mg

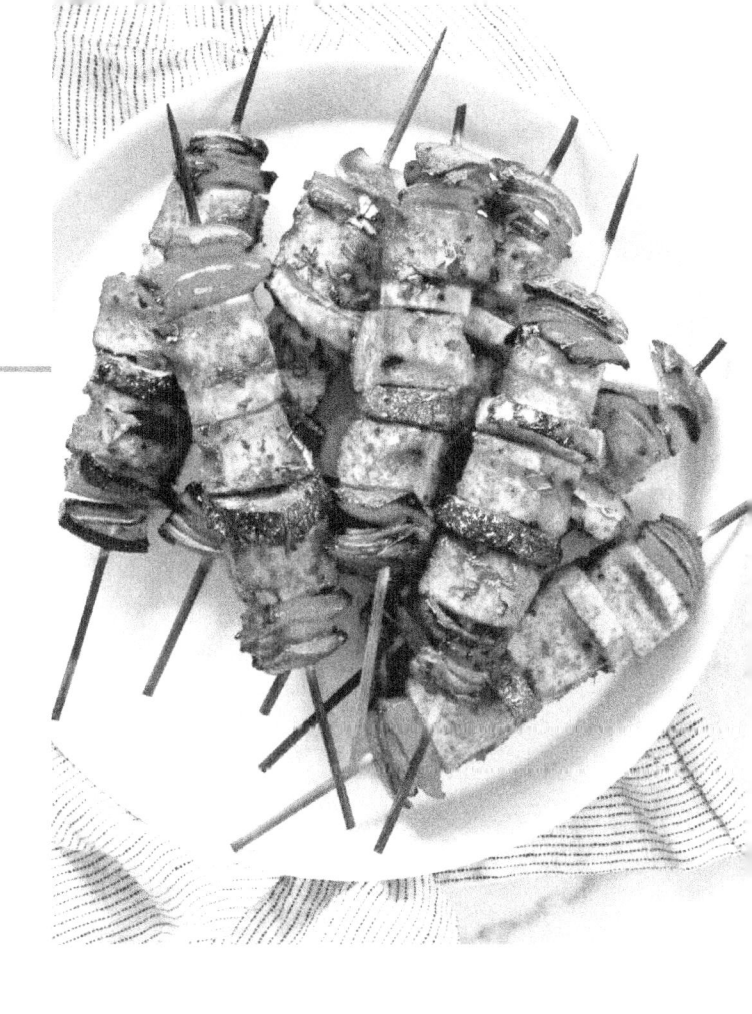

Grilled Chicken and Quinoa Salad

- **Preparation Time:** 15 minutes
- **Cooking Time:** 20 minutes
- **Servings:** 4

Ingredients:

- 2 boneless, skinless chicken breasts
- 1 cup quinoa
- 2 cups water
- 1 cup cherry tomatoes, halved
- 1 cucumber, diced
- 1/4 cup fresh parsley, chopped
- 2 tablespoons olive oil
- Juice of 1 lemon
- Black pepper to taste

Instructions:

1. Rinse quinoa under cold water. In a saucepan, combine quinoa and water. Bring to a boil, then reduce heat and simmer for 15 minutes. Let it cool.
2. Grill chicken breasts until fully cooked, about 6–7 minutes per side. Slice into strips.
3. In a large bowl, combine cooked quinoa, cherry tomatoes, cucumber, and parsley.
4. In a small bowl, whisk together olive oil, lemon juice, and black pepper.
5. Pour dressing over the salad and toss to combine. Top with grilled chicken slices.

Portion per Day: 1 serving

Nutritional Values (per serving):

- **Calories:** 350 kcal
- **Protein:** 30 g
- **Cholesterol:** 70 m
- **Carbohydrates:** 28 g
- **Fats:** 15 g
- **Fiber:** 5 g
- **Sodium:** 120 mg

Baked Cod with Lemon and Dill

- **Preparation Time:** 10 minutes
- **Cooking Time:** 15 minutes
- **Servings:** 4

Ingredients:

- 4 cod fillets (4 oz each)
- 2 tablespoons fresh lemon juice
- 1 tablespoon olive oil
- 2 teaspoons fresh dill, chopped
- 1 teaspoon garlic powder
- Black pepper to taste

Instructions:

1. Preheat oven to 375°F (190°C).
2. Place cod fillets in a baking dish.
3. In a small bowl, mix lemon juice, olive oil, dill, garlic powder, and black pepper.
4. Pour the mixture over the cod fillets.
5. Bake for 15 minutes or until fish flakes easily with a fork.

Portion per Day: 1 serving

Nutritional Values (per serving):

- **Calories:** 200 kcal
- **Protein:** 25 g
- **Carbohydrates:** 2 g
- **Fats:** 10 g
- **Fiber:** 0 g
- **Sodium:** 80 mg
- **Cholesterol:** 60 mg

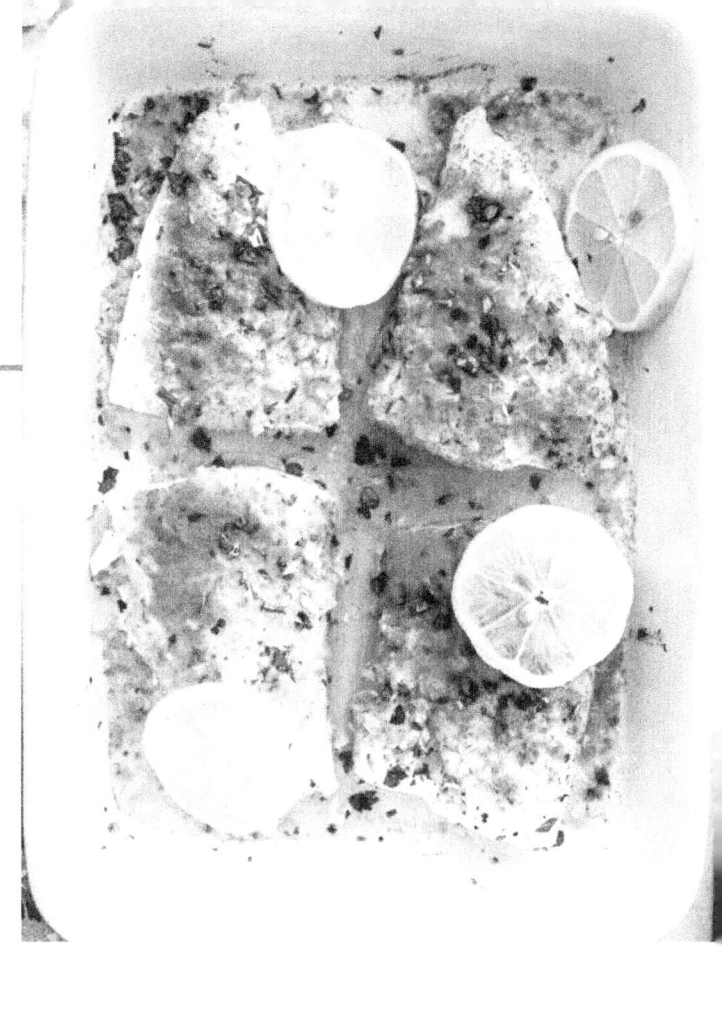

Chickpea and Avocado Lettuce Wraps

- **Preparation Time:** 15 minutes
- **Cooking Time:** 0 minutes
- **Servings:** 4

Ingredients:

- 1 can (15 oz) no-salt-added chickpeas, drained and rinsed
- 1 ripe avocado
- 1 tablespoon lemon juice
- 1/4 cup red onion, finely chopped
- 1/4 cup fresh cilantro, chopped
- 8 large lettuce leaves (e.g., romaine or butter lettuce)
- Black pepper to taste

Instructions:

1. In a bowl, mash chickpeas and avocado together until combined but still chunky.
2. Stir in lemon juice, red onion, cilantro, and black pepper.
3. Spoon the mixture into lettuce leaves and serve as wraps.

Portion per Day: 1 serving (2 wraps)

Nutritional Values (per serving):

- **Calories:** 250 kcal
- **Protein:** 10 g
- **Carbohydrates:** 20 g
- **Fats:** 15 g
- **Fiber:** 8 g
- **Sodium:** 90 mg
- **Cholesterol:** 0 mg

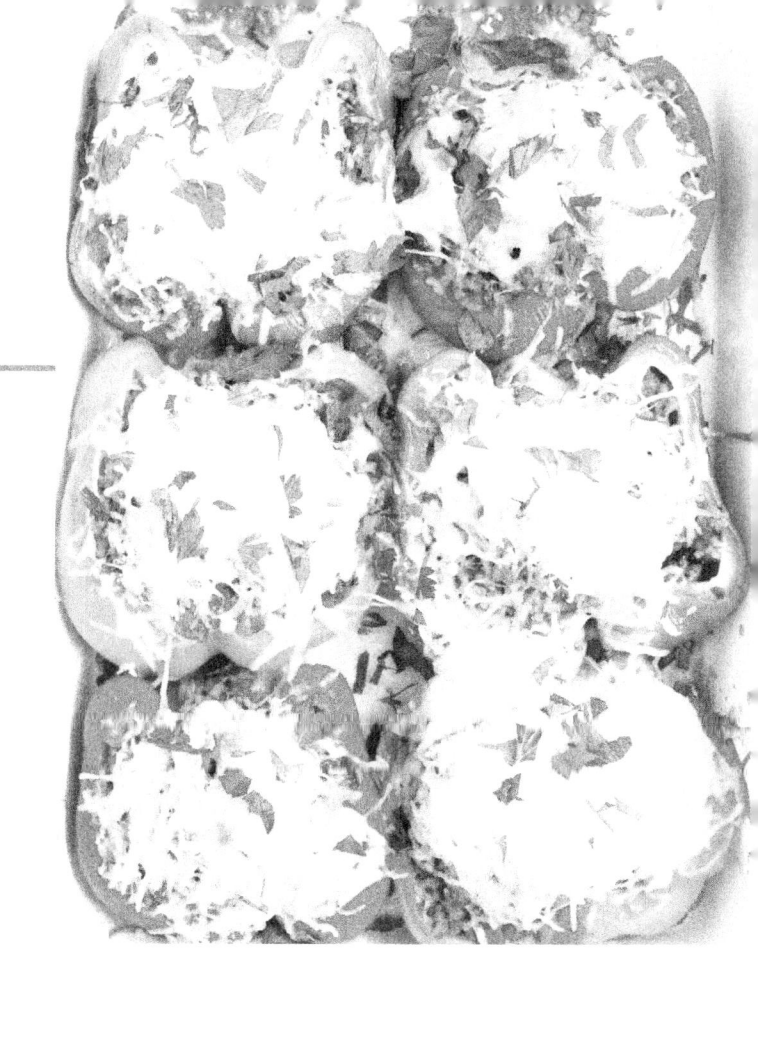

Turkey and Spinach Stuffed Bell Peppers

- **Preparation Time:** 20 minutes
- **Cooking Time:** 30 minutes
- **Servings:** 4

Ingredients:

- 4 large bell peppers, tops removed and seeds discarded
- 1 lb ground turkey (lean)
- 2 cups fresh spinach, chopped
- 1/2 cup cooked brown rice
- 1/2 cup no-salt-added tomato sauce
- 1 teaspoon dried basil
- 1 tablespoon olive oil
- Black pepper to taste

Instructions:

1. Preheat oven to 375°F (190°C).
2. In a skillet, heat olive oil over medium heat. Add ground turkey and cook until browned.
3. Stir in chopped spinach, cooked rice, tomato sauce, basil, and black pepper. Cook for 5 minutes.
4. Stuff the mixture into bell peppers and place them in a baking dish.
5. Cover with foil and bake for 30 minutes.

Portion per Day: 1 stuffed pepper

Nutritional Values (per serving):

- **Calories:** 300 kcal
- **Protein:** 25 g
- **Carbohydrates:** 20 g
- **Fats:** 12 g
- **Fiber:** 5 g
- **Sodium:** 100 mg
- **Cholesterol:** 70 mg

Tofu Stir-Fry with Brown Rice

- **Preparation Time:** 10 minutes
- **Cooking Time:** 15 minutes
- **Servings:** 2

Ingredients:

- 1 block firm tofu, cubed
- 1 tbsp sesame oil
- 1 cup mixed bell peppers
- 1 cup broccoli florets
- 2 tbsp low-sodium tamari
- 1 cup cooked brown rice

Instructions:

1. Sauté tofu in sesame oil until golden brown.
2. Add vegetables and stir-fry 5 minutes.
3. Stir in tamari and cook 2 more minutes. Serve with rice.

Portion per Day: 1 bowl

Nutritional Values (per serving):

- **Calories:** 390
- **Protein:** 25g
- **Carbohydrates:** 35g
- **Fats:** 18g
- **Fiber:** 6g
- **Sodium:** 140mg
- **Cholesterol:** 0mg

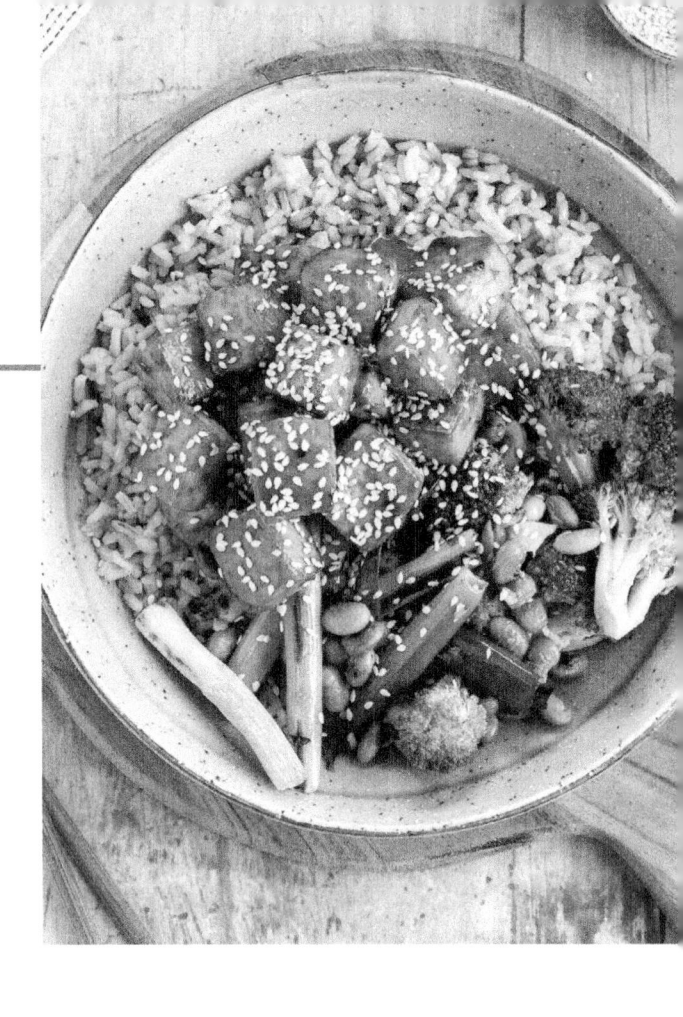

Sardine and Avocado Whole Grain Sandwich

- **Preparation Time:** 10 minutes
- **Cooking Time:** None
- **Servings:** 2

Ingredients:

- 1 can low-sodium sardines in water
- ½ avocado
- 4 slices whole grain bread
- 1 tbsp lemon juice
- Lettuce leaves

Instructions:

1. Mash sardines with avocado and lemon juice.
2. Spread on bread with lettuce.
3. Slice and serve as sandwiches.

Portion per Day: 1 sandwich

Nutritional Values (per serving):

- **Calories:** 350
- **Protein:** 22g
- **Carbohydrates:** 28g
- **Fats:** 20g
- **Fiber:** 5g
- **Sodium:** 130mg
- **Cholesterol:** 60mg

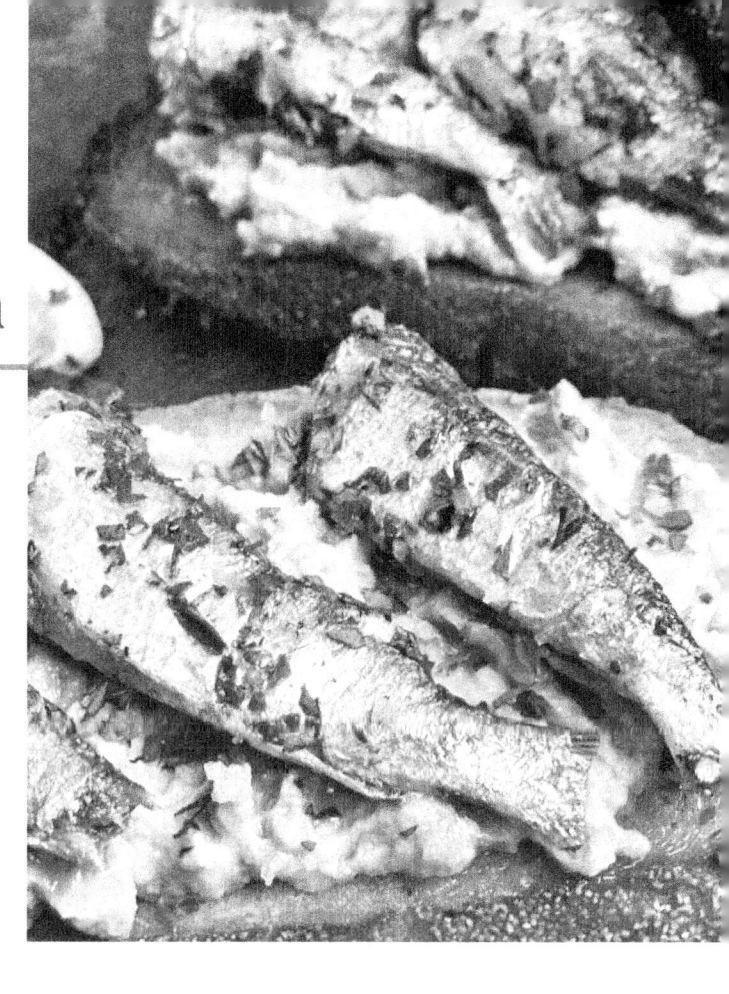

Grilled Chicken and Cucumber Wrap

- **Preparation Time:** 10 minutes
- **Cooking Time:** 10 minutes
- **Servings:** 2

Ingredients:

- 1 grilled chicken breast, sliced
- 1 cup chopped cucumber
- 2 tbsp plain Greek yogurt
- 1 tsp lemon juice
- 2 whole wheat low-sodium wraps

Instructions:

1. Mix yogurt with lemon juice for sauce.
2. Layer chicken and cucumber in wrap.
3. Drizzle sauce, roll, and slice.

Portion per Day: 1 wrap

Nutritional Values (per serving):

- **Calories:** 320
- **Protein:** 29g
- **Carbohydrates:** 22g
- **Fats:** 11g
- **Fiber:** 4g
- **Sodium:** 110mg
- **Cholesterol:** 55mg

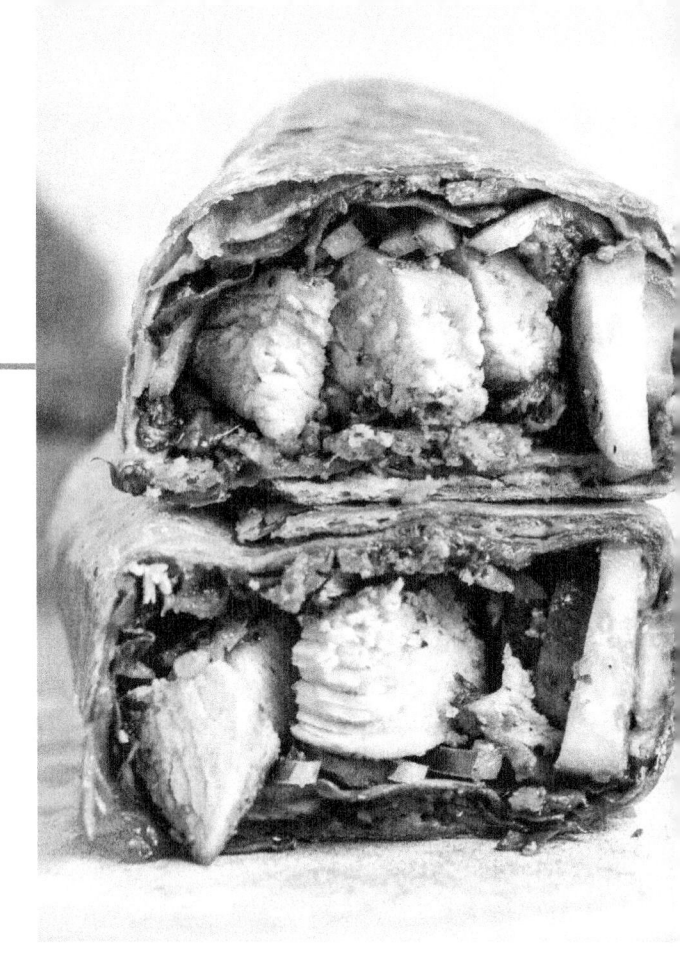

Red Lentil and Carrot Soup

- **Preparation Time:** 10 minutes
- **Cooking Time:** 25 minutes
- **Servings:** 3

Ingredients:

- ¾ cup red lentils
- 1 cup chopped carrots
- ½ onion, chopped
- 2 garlic cloves, minced
- 4 cups water
- 1 tbsp olive oil
- ½ tsp cumin

Instructions:

1. Sauté onion and garlic in olive oil for 5 minutes.
2. Add carrots, lentils, cumin, and water. Simmer 20 minutes.
3. Blend if preferred for smoother texture.

Portion per Day: 1.5 cups

Nutritional Values (per serving):

- **Calories:** 290
- **Protein:** 19g
- **Carbohydrates:** 32g
- **Fats:** 8g
- **Fiber:** 9g
- **Sodium:** 80mg
- **Cholesterol:** 0mg

Edamame and Barley Power Bowl

- **Preparation Time:** 10 minutes
- **Cooking Time:** 30 minutes
- **Servings:** 2

Ingredients:

- 1 cup cooked barley
- 1 cup shelled edamame (cooked)
- ½ cup diced cucumber
- 1 tbsp olive oil
- 1 tbsp lemon juice
- 1 tbsp chopped fresh mint

Instructions:

1. Cook barley until tender. Let cool.
2. Toss all ingredients together in a bowl.
3. Serve chilled or at room temperature.

Portion per Day: 1 bowl

Nutritional Values (per serving):

- **Calories:** 340
- **Protein:** 22g
- **Carbohydrates:** 30g
- **Fats:** 14g
- **Fiber:** 7g
- **Sodium:** 90mg
- **Cholesterol:** 0mg

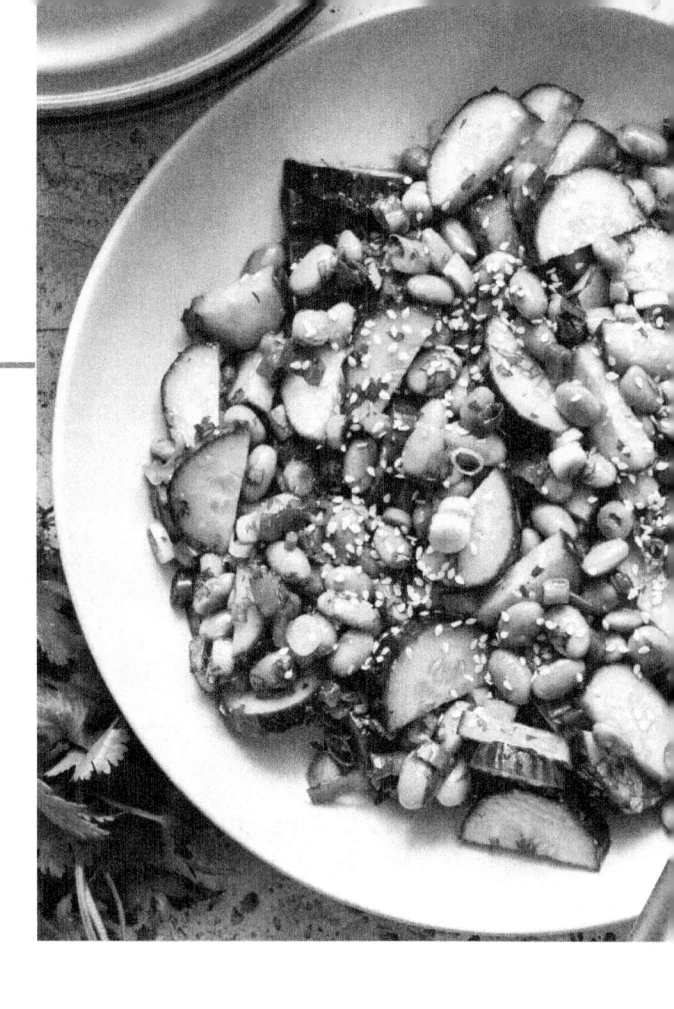

Tempeh and Veggie Stir Fry

- **Preparation Time:** 10 minutes
- **Cooking Time:** 15 minutes
- **Servings:** 2

Ingredients:

- 1 cup tempeh, cubed
- 1 cup mixed bell peppers
- ½ cup snap peas
- 1 tbsp olive oil
- 1 tbsp low-sodium tamari
- 1 tsp grated ginger

Instructions:

1. Sauté tempeh in olive oil for 5 minutes.
2. Add vegetables and ginger, stir-fry for 7 minutes.
3. Add tamari and cook 2 more minutes.

Portion per Day: 1 bowl

Nutritional Values (per serving):

- **Calories:** 360
- **Protein:** 24g
- **Carbohydrates:** 18g
- **Fats:** 20g
- **Fiber:** 5g
- **Sodium:** 110mg
- **Cholesterol:** 0mg

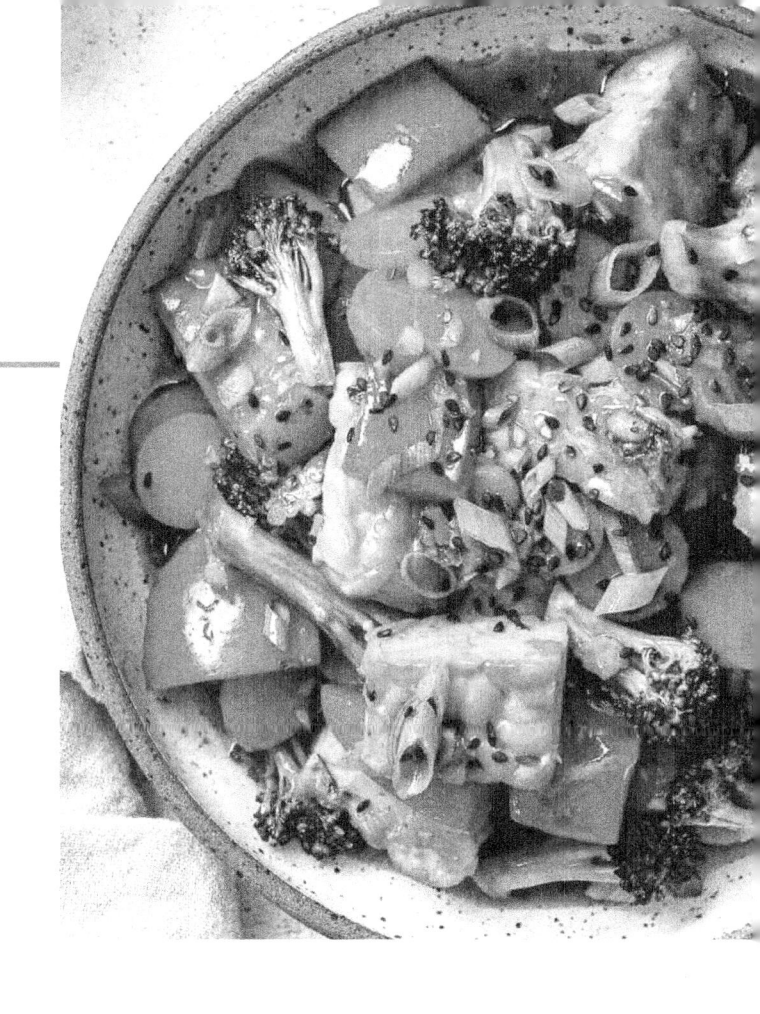

Baked Falafel with Cucumber Yogurt Dip

- **Preparation Time:** 15 minutes
- **Cooking Time:** 25 minutes
- **Servings:** 3

Ingredients:

- 1 cup cooked chickpeas
- 1 garlic clove
- 2 tbsp oat flour
- 1 tbsp fresh parsley
- ½ tsp cumin
- 2 tbsp Greek yogurt
- 2 tbsp grated cucumber

Instructions:

1. Blend chickpeas, garlic, parsley, cumin, and oat flour into a dough.
2. Form into patties, bake at 375°F for 25 minutes.
3. Mix yogurt and cucumber for dip.

Portion per Day: 2 falafel + 1 tbsp dip

Nutritional Values (per serving):

- **Calories:** 290
- **Protein:** 16g
- **Carbohydrates:** 25g
- **Fats:** 12g
- **Fiber:** 7g
- **Sodium:** 85mg
- **Cholesterol:** 5mg

CHAPTER 06
DINNERS

As the final meal of the day, dinner offers a crucial opportunity to gently support your liver, particularly for seniors managing cirrhosis. More than just satisfying evening hunger, a thoughtfully prepared dinner should aid the liver's overnight functions. The right choices can help regulate metabolism, stabilize blood sugar, minimize inflammation, and prevent nighttime discomforts like bloating or fluid retention.

This collection features dinner recipes carefully chosen for their deliciousness, simplicity, and supportive qualities. Each recipe prioritizes low-fat content to ease the liver's workload, ample lean protein to maintain muscle health, and a wealth of fiber and micronutrients to encourage smooth digestion. Sodium is strictly controlled, and processed ingredients, red meat, and excess fats are intentionally excluded. Explore a diverse selection of meals, from tender baked fish with vibrant vegetables to flavorful tofu stir-fries, nourishing grain bowls, hearty veggie-filled stews, and light, plant-forward options.

Designed for convenience, these recipes utilize everyday ingredients and straightforward steps, making them ideal for seniors, caregivers, and anyone seeking nutritious simplicity. Whether you dine early or late, solo or with loved ones, this section provides a complete set of reliable meals tailored to your body's needs. Eliminate the guesswork of what's safe and nutritious and rediscover the pleasure of enjoying a supportive and delicious dinner.

Lemon Herb Grilled Chicken with Steamed Broccoli

- **Preparation Time:** 10 minutes
- **Cooking Time:** 15 minutes
- **Servings:** 2

Ingredients:

- 2 skinless, boneless chicken breasts
- Juice of 1 lemon
- 1 tablespoon olive oil
- 1 teaspoon dried oregano
- 2 cups broccoli florets
- Salt and pepper to taste

Instructions:

1. Marinate chicken breasts in lemon juice, olive oil, oregano, salt, and pepper for 10 minutes.
2. Grill chicken over medium heat for 6-7 minutes on each side until fully cooked.
3. Steam broccoli florets for 5 minutes until tender.
4. Serve grilled chicken alongside steamed broccoli.

Portion per Day: 1 serving

Nutritional Values (per serving):

- **Calories:** 250 kcal
- **Protein:** 35 g
- **Carbohydrates:** 8 g
- **Fats:** 8 g
- **Fiber:** 3 g
- **Sodium:** 150 mg
- **Cholesterol:** 85 mg

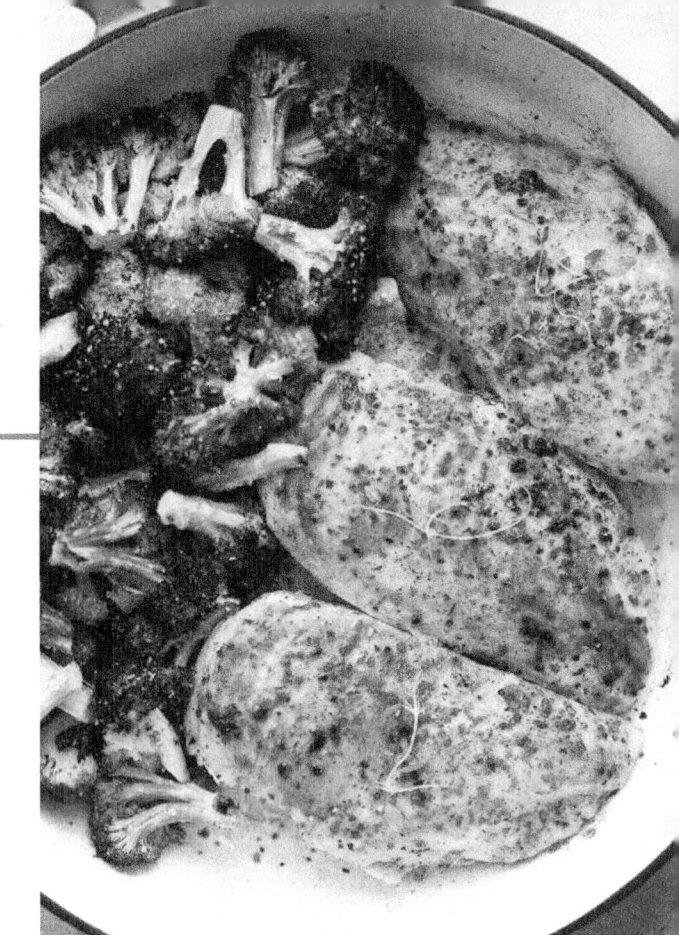

Baked Cod with Quinoa and Asparagus

- **Preparation Time:** 10 minutes
- **Cooking Time:** 20 minutes
- **Servings:** 2

Ingredients:

- 2 cod fillets (4 oz each)
- 1 cup cooked quinoa
- 1 bunch asparagus, trimmed
- 1 tablespoon olive oil
- 1 teaspoon garlic powder
- Juice of 1/2 lemon
- Salt and pepper to taste

Instructions:

1. Preheat oven to 375°F (190°C).
2. Place cod fillets on a baking sheet, drizzle with olive oil, lemon juice, garlic powder, salt, and pepper.
3. Bake for 15-20 minutes until fish flakes easily.
4. Steam asparagus for 5 minutes until tender.
5. Serve baked cod with quinoa and steamed asparagus.

Portion per Day: 1 serving

Nutritional Values (per serving):

- **Calories:** 320 kcal
- **Protein:** 30 g
- **Carbohydrates:** 25 g
- **Fats:** 10 g
- **Fiber:** 5 g
- **Sodium:** 140 mg
- **Cholesterol:** 60 mg

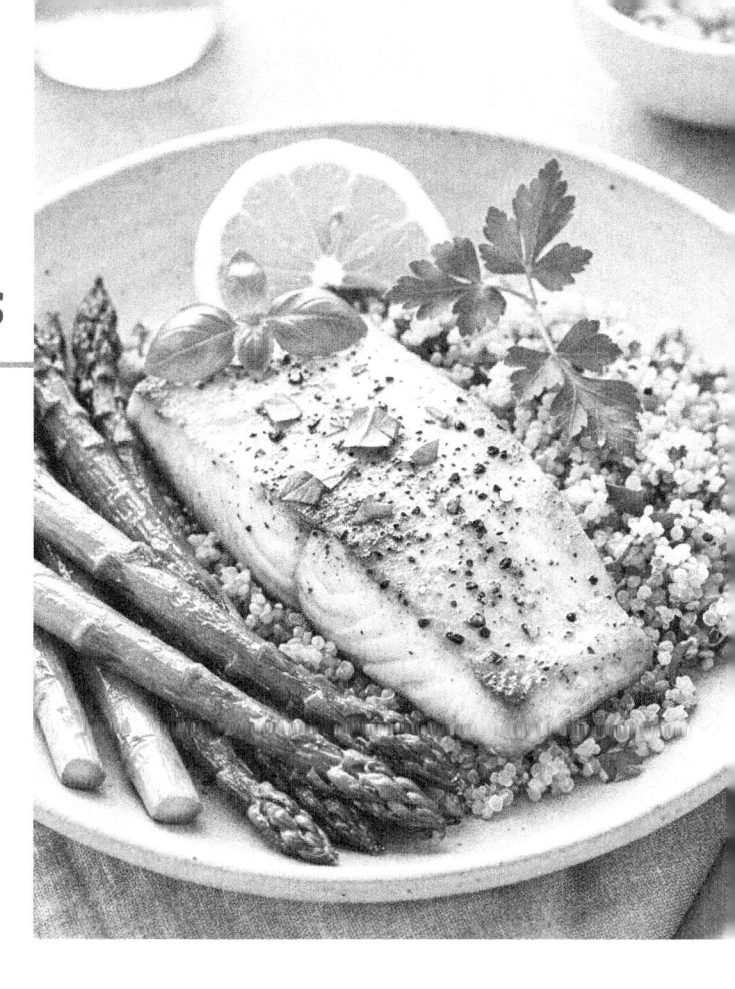

Quinoa and Black Bean Stuffed Peppers

- **Preparation Time:** 20 minutes
- **Cooking Time:** 30 minutes
- **Servings:** 2

Ingredients:

- 2 large bell peppers, halved and seeded
- 1 cup cooked quinoa
- 1 cup canned black beans, rinsed
- 1/2 cup corn kernels
- 1/2 cup diced tomatoes
- 1 teaspoon cumin
- 1 teaspoon chili powder
- Salt and pepper to taste

Instructions:

1. Preheat oven to 375°F (190°C).
2. In a bowl, mix quinoa, black beans, corn, tomatoes, cumin, chili powder, salt, and pepper.
3. Fill bell pepper halves with the mixture.
4. Place stuffed peppers in a baking dish, cover with foil, and bake for 30 minutes.
5. Serve warm.

Portion per Day: 1 stuffed pepper half

Nutritional Values (per serving):

- **Calories:** 310 kcal
- **Protein:** 15 g
- **Carbohydrates:** 40 g
- **Fats:** 8 g
- **Fiber:** 10 g
- **Sodium:** 180 mg
- **Cholesterol:** 0 mg

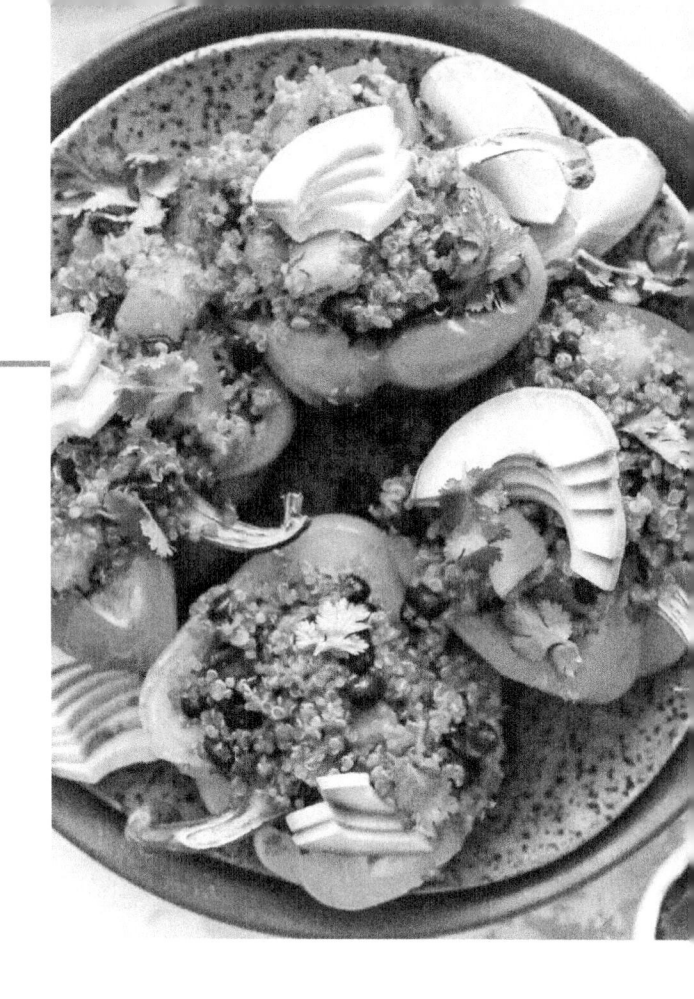

Grilled Salmon with Spinach & Brown Rice

- **Preparation Time:** 10 minutes
- **Cooking Time:** 15 minutes
- **Servings:** 2

Ingredients:

- 2 salmon fillets (4 oz each)
- 2 cups fresh spinach
- 1 cup cooked brown rice
- 1 tablespoon olive oil
- Juice of 1/2 lemon
- Salt and pepper to taste

Instructions:

1. Preheat grill to medium heat.
2. Season salmon with lemon juice, salt, and pepper.
3. Grill salmon for 6-7 minutes on each side until cooked through.
4. In a pan, sauté spinach in olive oil until wilted.
5. Serve grilled salmon with sautéed spinach and brown rice.

Portion per Day: 1 serving

Nutritional Values (per serving):

- **Calories:** 350 kcal
- **Protein:** 30 g
- **Carbohydrates:** 30 g
- **Fats:** 15 g
- **Fiber:** 5 g
- **Sodium:** 120 mg
- **Cholesterol:** 70 mg

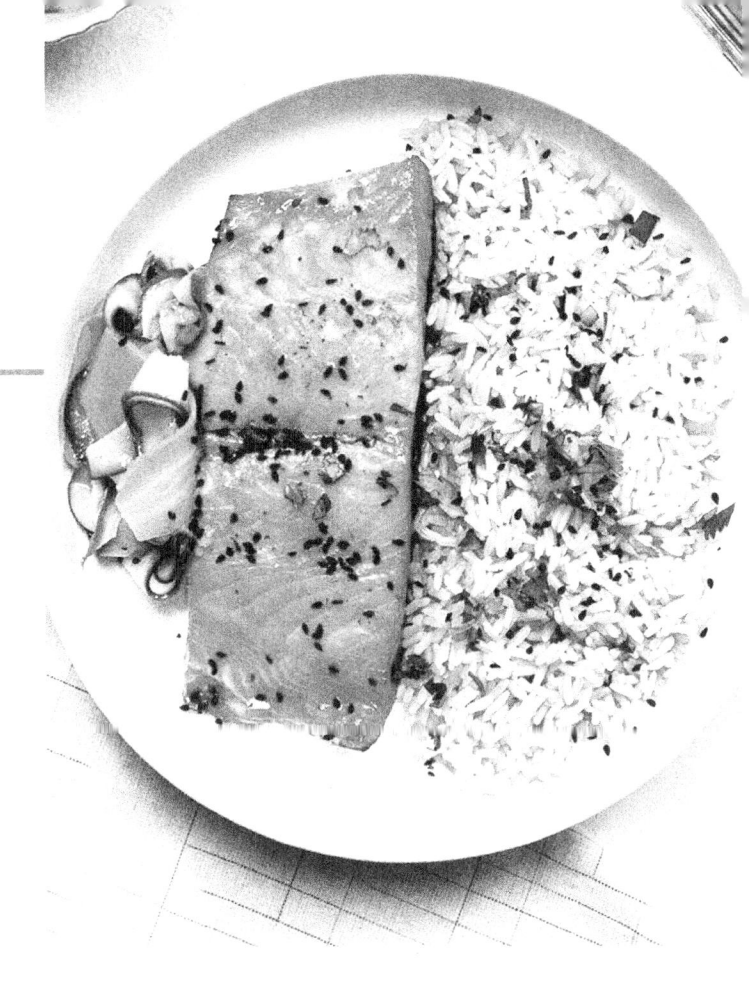

Baked Tilapia with Lemon and Herbs

- **Preparation Time:** 10 minutes
- **Cooking Time:** 15 minutes
- **Servings:** 2

Ingredients:

- 2 tilapia fillets (4 oz each)
- 1 tablespoon olive oil
- Juice of 1 lemon
- 1 teaspoon dried oregano
- 1 teaspoon garlic powder
- Salt and pepper to taste

Instructions:

1. Preheat oven to 375°F (190°C).
2. Place tilapia fillets on a baking sheet lined with parchment paper.
3. Drizzle olive oil and lemon juice over the fillets.
4. Sprinkle with oregano, garlic powder, salt, and pepper.
5. Bake for 15 minutes or until fish flakes easily with a fork.

Portion per Day: 1 fillet

Nutritional Values (per serving):

- **Calories:** 220 kcal
- **Protein:** 30 g
- **Carbohydrates:** 2 g
- **Fats:** 10 g
- **Fiber:** 0 g
- **Sodium:** 100 mg
- **Cholesterol:** 60 mg

Quinoa and Vegetable Stir-Fry

- **Preparation Time:** 15 minutes
- **Cooking Time:** 10 minutes
- **Servings:** 2

Ingredients:

- 1 cup cooked quinoa
- 1 cup mixed vegetables (e.g., bell peppers, broccoli, carrots)
- 1 tablespoon olive oil
- 1 tablespoon low-sodium soy sauce
- 1 teaspoon grated ginger
- 1 clove garlic, minced

Instructions:

1. Heat olive oil in a large skillet over medium heat.
2. Add garlic and ginger; sauté for 1 minute.
3. Add mixed vegetables; stir-fry for 5 minutes until tender-crisp.
4. Stir in cooked quinoa and soy sauce; cook for an additional 2 minutes.
5. Serve hot.

Portion per Day: 1 serving

Nutritional Values (per serving):

- **Calories:** 300 kcal
- **Protein:** 12 g
- **Carbohydrates:** 40 g
- **Fats:** 10 g
- **Fiber:** 6 g
- **Sodium:** 150 mg
- **Cholesterol:** 0 mg

Grilled Chicken Salad with Avocado

- **Preparation Time:** 15 minutes
- **Cooking Time:** 10 minutes
- **Servings:** 2

Ingredients:

- 2 skinless, boneless chicken breasts
- 4 cups mixed salad greens
- 1 avocado, sliced
- 1/2 cup cherry tomatoes, halved
- 1 tablespoon olive oil
- Juice of 1 lemon
- Salt and pepper to taste

Instructions:

1. Season chicken breasts with salt and pepper.
2. Grill chicken over medium heat for 5-6 minutes on each side until cooked through.
3. In a large bowl, combine salad greens, avocado slices, and cherry tomatoes.
4. Slice grilled chicken and add to the salad.
5. Drizzle with olive oil and lemon juice before serving.

Portion per Day: 1 serving

Nutritional Values (per serving):

- **Calories:** 350 kcal
- **Protein:** 30 g
- **Carbohydrates:** 10 g
- **Fats:** 20 g
- **Fiber:** 7 g
- **Sodium:** 120 mg
- **Cholesterol:** 70 mg

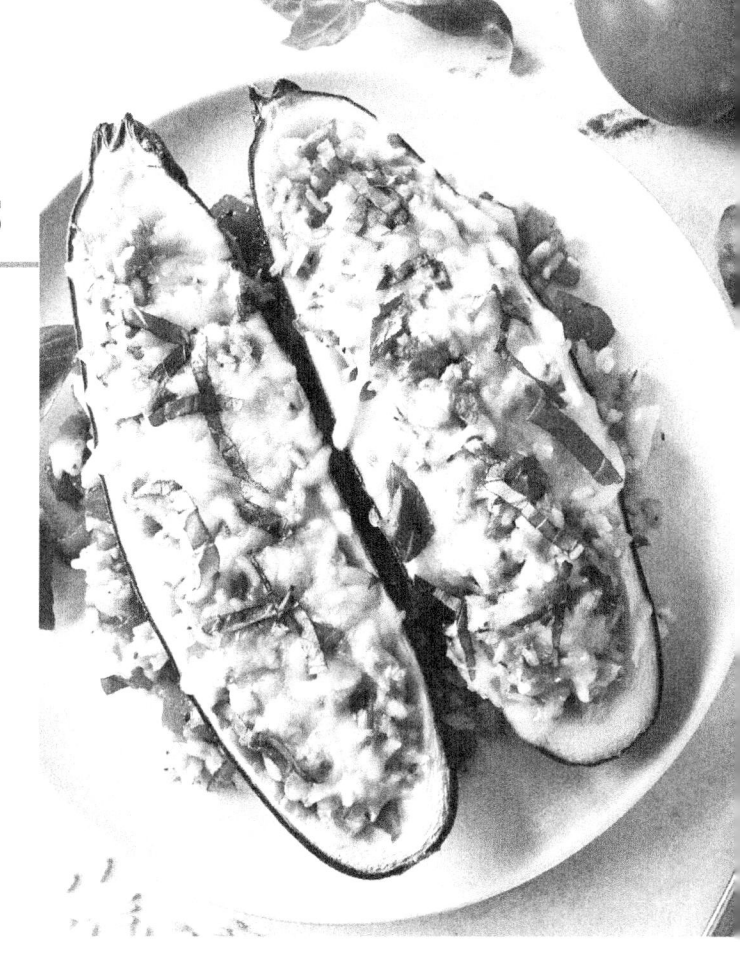

Stuffed Zucchini Boats

- **Preparation Time:** 15 minutes
- **Cooking Time:** 20 minutes
- **Servings:** 2

Ingredients:

- 2 medium zucchinis, halved lengthwise and seeds scooped out
- 1 cup cooked brown rice
- 1/2 cup diced tomatoes
- 1/4 cup chopped onions
- 1/4 cup chopped bell peppers
- 1 tablespoon olive oil
- 1 teaspoon Italian seasoning
- Salt and pepper to taste

Instructions:

1. Preheat oven to 375°F (190°C).
2. In a skillet, heat olive oil over medium heat.
3. Sauté onions and bell peppers until softened.
4. Add diced tomatoes, cooked brown rice, Italian seasoning, salt, and pepper; cook for 5 minutes.
5. Fill zucchini halves with the rice mixture.
6. Place stuffed zucchinis on a baking sheet and bake for 20 minutes.
7. Serve warm.

Portion per Day: 1 zucchini boat

Nutritional Values (per serving):

- **Calories:** 250 kcal
- **Protein:** 6 g
- **Carbohydrates:** 35 g
- **Fats:** 10 g
- **Fiber:** 5 g
- **Sodium:** 90 mg
- **Cholesterol:** 0 mg

Quinoa and Chickpea Salad

- **Preparation Time:** 15 minutes
- **Cooking Time:** 15 minutes
- **Servings:** 2

Ingredients:

- 1 cup cooked quinoa
- 1 cup canned chickpeas, rinsed and drained
- 1/2 cucumber, diced
- 1/2 red bell pepper, diced
- 1/4 cup red onion, finely chopped
- 2 tablespoons olive oil
- Juice of 1 lemon
- 1 tablespoon chopped fresh parsley
- Salt and pepper to taste

Instructions:

1. In a large bowl, combine cooked quinoa, chickpeas, cucumber, bell pepper, and red onion.
2. In a small bowl, whisk together olive oil, lemon juice, parsley, salt, and pepper.
3. Pour the dressing over the salad and toss to combine.
4. Refrigerate for at least 30 minutes before serving to allow flavors to meld.

Portion per Day: 1 serving

Nutritional Values (per serving):

- **Calories:** 320 kcal
- **Protein:** 12 g
- **Carbohydrates:** 40 g
- **Fats:** 12 g
- **Fiber:** 8 g
- **Sodium:** 180 mg
- **Cholesterol:** 0 mg

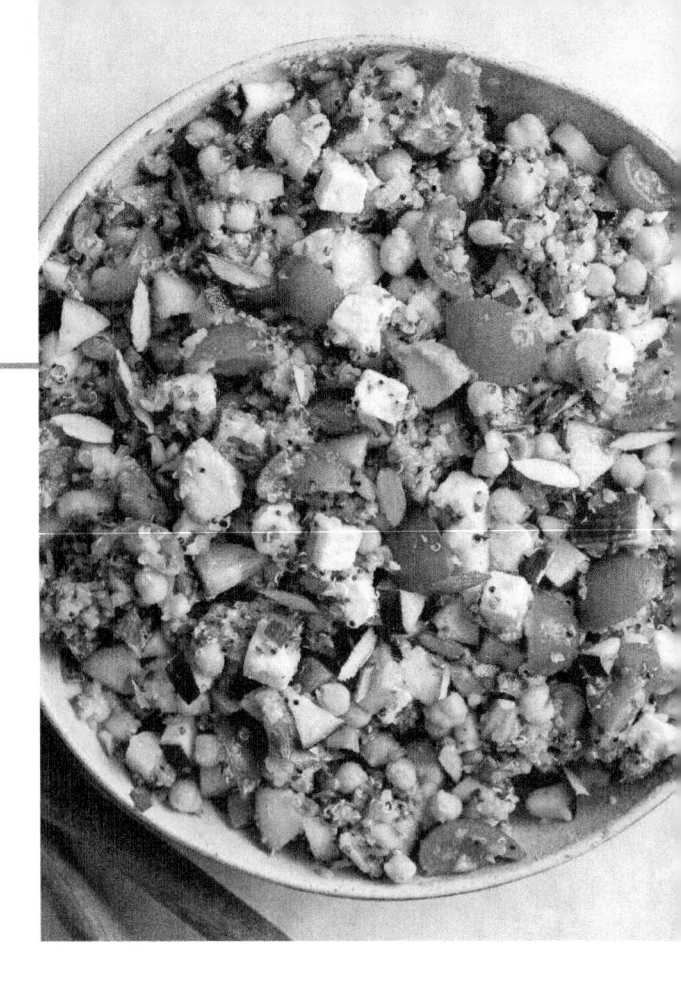

Grilled Portobello Mushrooms with Brown Rice

- **Preparation Time:** 10 minutes
- **Cooking Time:** 20 minutes
- **Servings:** 2

Ingredients:

- 2 large portobello mushroom caps
- 1 tablespoon balsamic vinegar
- 1 tablespoon olive oil
- 1 teaspoon dried thyme
- 1 cup cooked brown rice
- 1 cup steamed green beans
- Salt and pepper to taste

Instructions:

1. In a small bowl, mix balsamic vinegar, olive oil, thyme, salt, and pepper.
2. Brush the mixture onto both sides of the mushroom caps.
3. Grill mushrooms over medium heat for 5-7 minutes on each side until tender.
4. Serve grilled mushrooms over brown rice with a side of steamed green beans.

Portion per Day: 1 serving

Nutritional Values (per serving):

- **Calories:** 300 kcal
- **Protein:** 8 g
- **Carbohydrates:** 40 g
- **Fats:** 10 g
- **Fiber:** 6 g
- **Sodium:** 150 mg
- **Cholesterol:** 0 mg

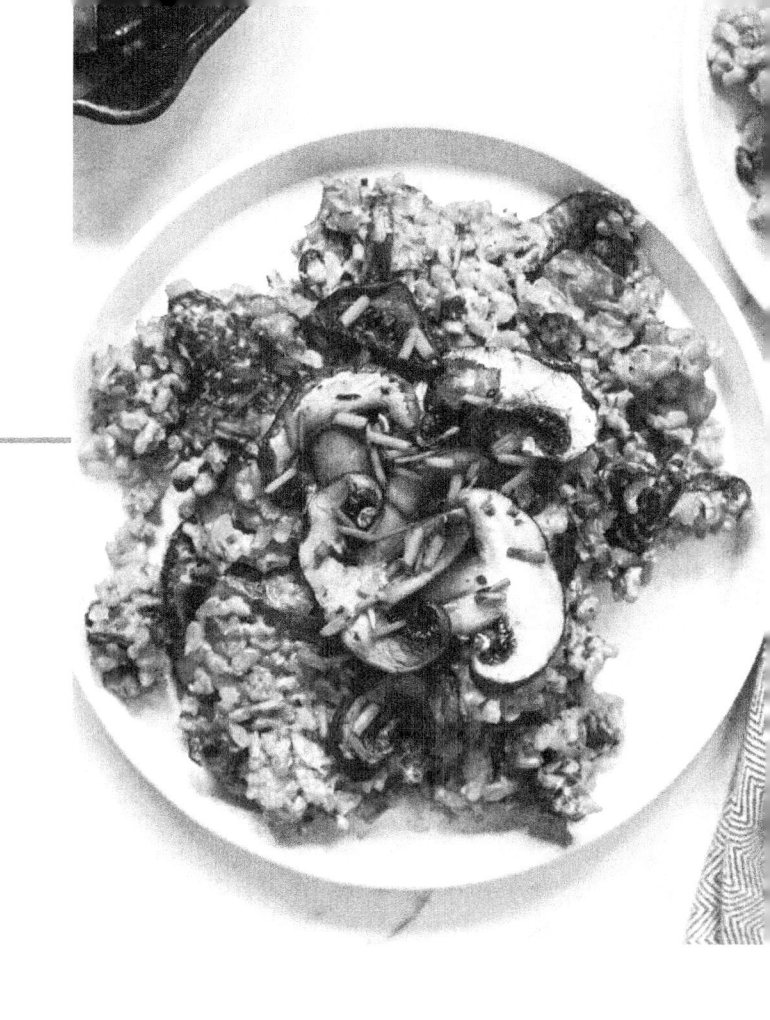

Grilled Turkey Burger with Avocado Spread

- **Preparation Time:** 10 minutes
- **Cooking Time:** 15 minutes
- **Servings:** 2

Ingredients:

- 8 oz ground turkey breast (lean)
- 1/2 teaspoon garlic powder
- 1/2 teaspoon onion powder
- 1/4 teaspoon black pepper
- 1 avocado, mashed
- Juice of 1/2 lemon
- 2 whole-grain burger buns
- Lettuce leaves and tomato slices for topping

Instructions:

1. In a bowl, mix ground turkey with garlic powder, onion powder, and black pepper. Form into two patties.
2. Grill patties over medium heat for 6-7 minutes on each side until cooked through.
3. In a separate bowl, combine mashed avocado with lemon juice to make the spread.
4. Toast the burger buns lightly.
5. Assemble the burgers by spreading avocado mixture on the buns, adding the turkey patty, lettuce, and tomato slices.

Portion per Day: 1 burger

Nutritional Values (per serving):

- **Calories:** 350 kcal
- **Protein:** 30 g
- **Carbohydrates:** 25 g
- **Fats:** 15 g
- **Fiber:** 5 g
- **Sodium:** 300 mg
- **Cholesterol:** 70 mg

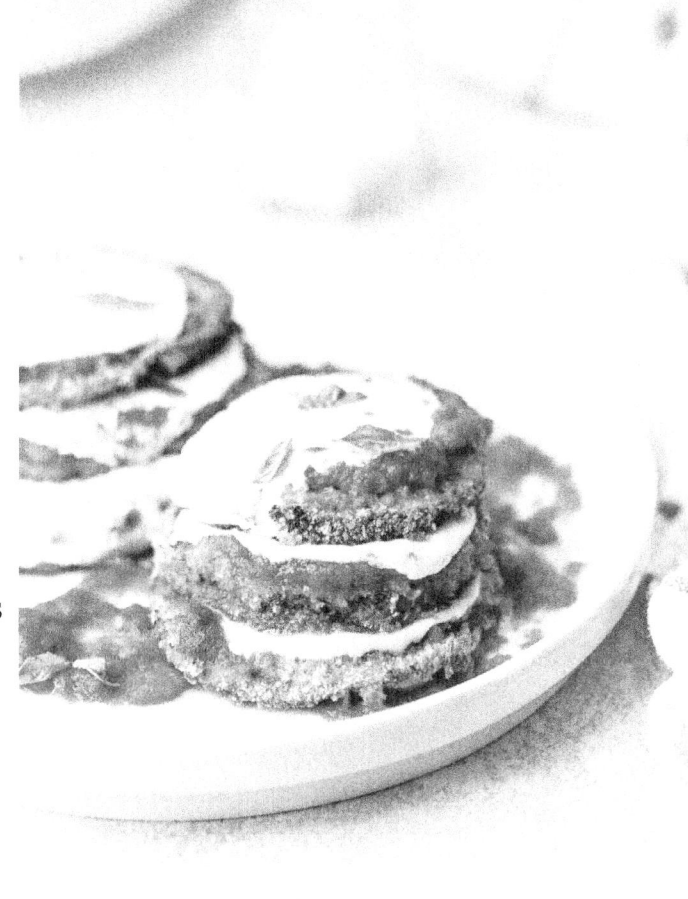

Baked Eggplant Parmesan

- **Preparation Time:** 15 minutes
- **Cooking Time:** 25 minutes
- **Servings:** 2

Ingredients:

- 1 medium eggplant, sliced into 1/2-inch rounds
- 1 cup whole wheat breadcrumbs
- 1/2 cup egg whites
- 1 cup low-sodium marinara sauce
- 1/2 cup shredded part-skim mozzarella cheese
- 1 tablespoon olive oil
- Fresh basil leaves for garnish

Instructions:

1. Preheat oven to 375°F (190°C).
2. Dip eggplant slices into egg whites, then coat with breadcrumbs.
3. Place coated eggplant slices on a baking sheet lined with parchment paper. Drizzle with olive oil.
4. Bake for 20 minutes, flipping halfway through.
5. Top each slice with marinara sauce and mozzarella cheese. Return to oven and bake for an additional 5 minutes until cheese melts.
6. Garnish with fresh basil before serving.

Portion per Day: 2-3 slices

Nutritional Values (per serving):

- **Calories:** 300 kcal
- **Protein:** 15 g
- **Carbohydrates:** 35 g
- **Fats:** 10 g
- **Fiber:** 7 g
- **Sodium:** 250 mg
- **Cholesterol:** 20 mg

Shrimp and Vegetable Stir-Fry

- **Preparation Time:** 10 minutes
- **Cooking Time:** 10 minutes
- **Servings:** 2

Ingredients:

- 8 oz shrimp, peeled and deveined
- 1 cup broccoli florets
- 1 bell pepper, sliced
- 1 carrot, julienned
- 2 tablespoons low-sodium soy sauce
- 1 tablespoon sesame oil
- 1 teaspoon grated ginger
- 2 cloves garlic, minced

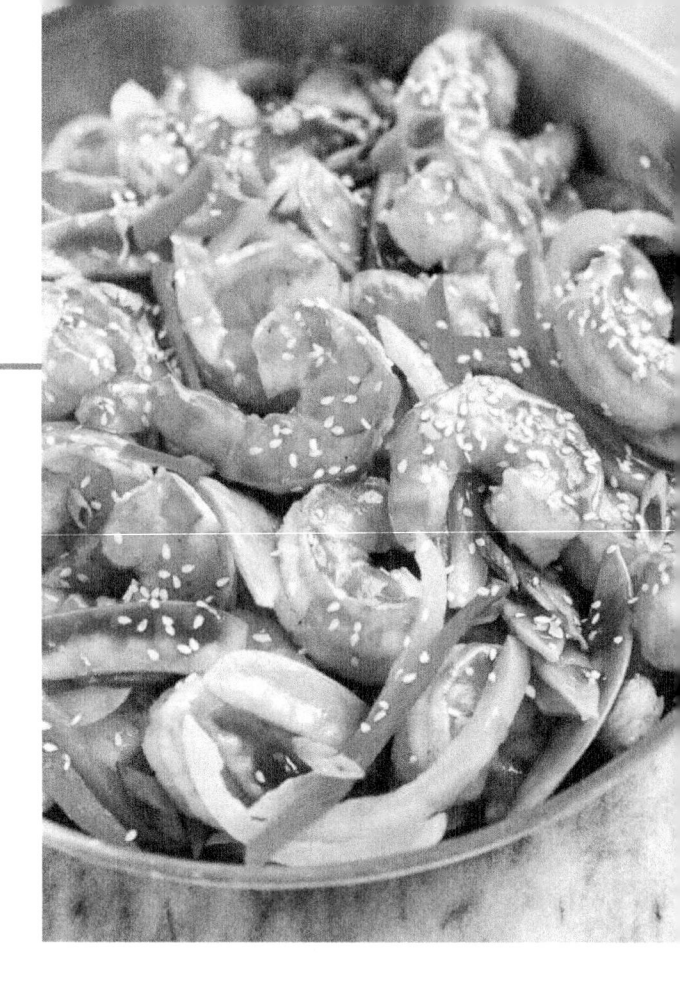

Instructions:

1. Heat sesame oil in a wok or large skillet over medium-high heat.
2. Add garlic and ginger; sauté for 1 minute.
3. Add shrimp and cook until pink, about 3-4 minutes. Remove and set aside.
4. Add vegetables to the skillet and stir-fry for 5 minutes until tender-crisp.
5. Return shrimp to the skillet, add soy sauce, and stir to combine. Cook for an additional 2 minutes.
6. Serve hot.

Portion per Day: 1 serving

Nutritional Values (per serving):

- **Calories:** 280 kcal
- **Protein:** 25 g
- **Carbohydrates:** 15 g
- **Fats:** 12 g
- **Fiber:** 4 g
- **Sodium:** 220 mg
- **Cholesterol:** 150 mg

Zucchini Noodles with Pesto and Cherry Tomatoes

- **Preparation Time:** 15 minutes
- **Cooking Time:** 5 minutes
- **Servings:** 2

Ingredients:

- 2 medium zucchinis, spiralized into noodles
- 1 cup cherry tomatoes, halved
- 2 tablespoons homemade basil pesto (made with olive oil, basil, garlic, and pine nuts)
- 1 tablespoon olive oil
- Salt and pepper to taste

Instructions:

1. In a large skillet, heat olive oil over medium heat.
2. Add zucchini noodles and sauté for 2-3 minutes until slightly tender.
3. Add cherry tomatoes and cook for another 2 minutes.
4. Remove from heat and toss with basil pesto.
5. Season with salt and pepper before serving.

Portion per Day: 1 serving

Nutritional Values (per serving):

- **Calories:** 250 kcal
- **Protein:** 6 g
- **Carbohydrates:** 15 g
- **Fats:** 20 g
- **Fiber:** 4 g
- **Sodium:** 150 mg
- **Cholesterol:** 0 mg

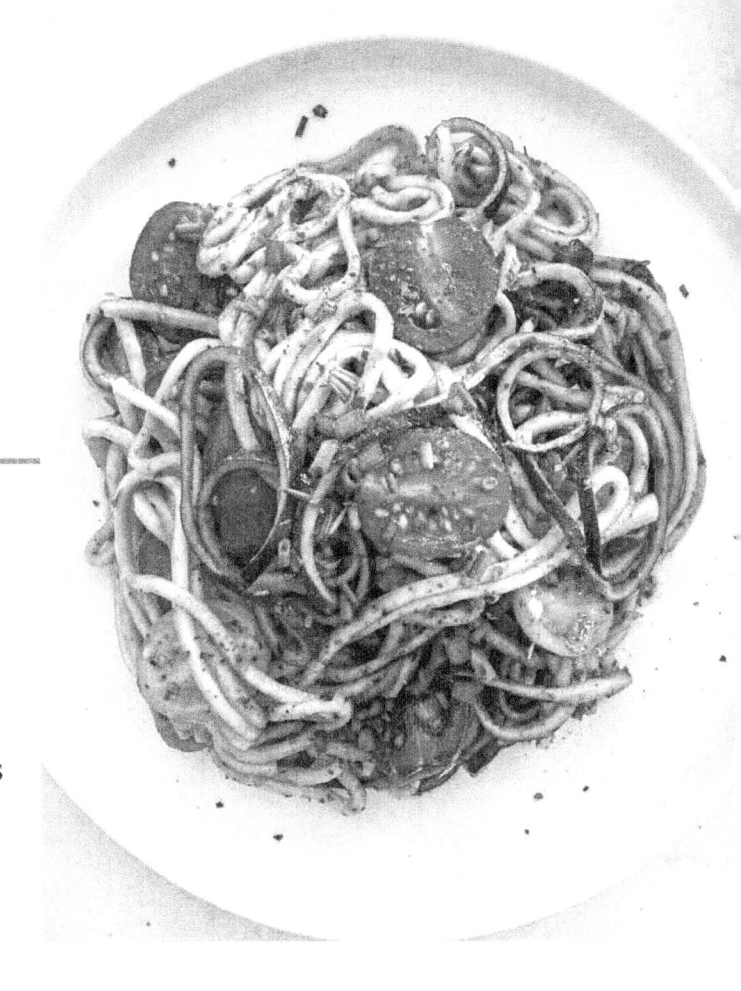

Cauliflower and Chickpea Curry

- **Preparation Time:** 10 minutes
- **Cooking Time:** 25 minutes
- **Servings:** 3

Ingredients:

- 2 cups cauliflower florets
- 1 cup canned low-sodium chickpeas, rinsed
- 1 small onion, diced
- 1 tsp grated ginger
- 1 garlic clove, minced
- 1 tsp turmeric
- 1 tbsp olive oil
- 1 cup unsweetened coconut milk

Instructions:

1. Sauté onion, garlic, and ginger in oil for 5 minutes.
2. Add turmeric, cauliflower, chickpeas, and coconut milk.
3. Simmer for 20 minutes until tender.

Portion per Day: 1 bowl (approx. 1.5 cups)

Nutritional Values (per serving):

- **Calories:** 330
- **Protein:** 14g
- **Carbohydrates:** 28g
- **Fats:** 18g
- **Fiber:** 9g
- **Sodium:** 95mg
- **Cholesterol:** 0mg

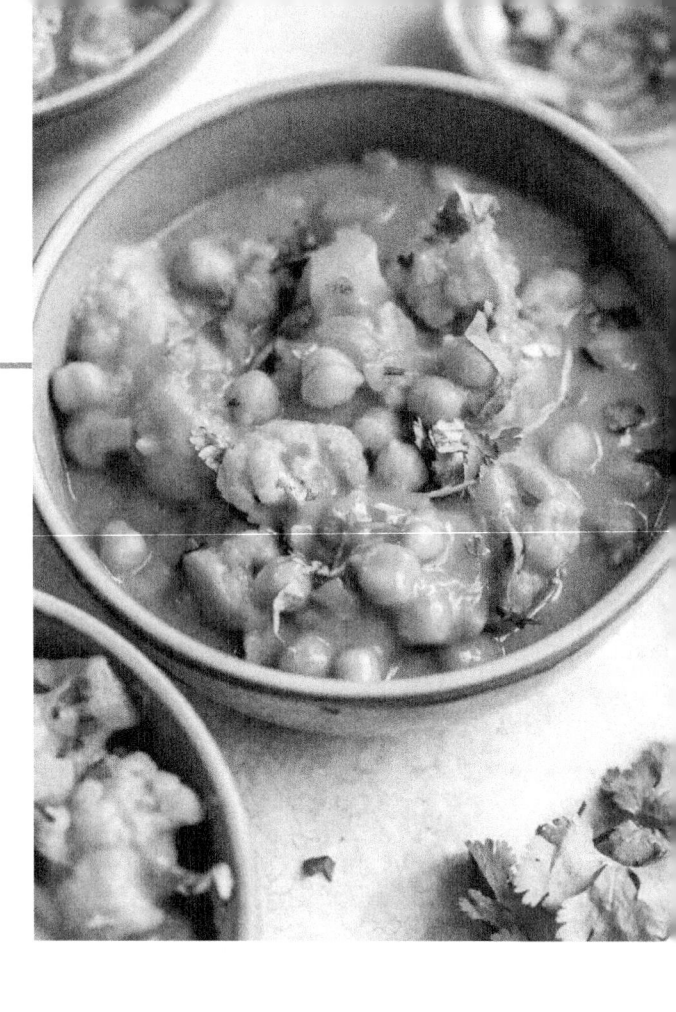

Seared Scallops with Spinach and Millet

- **Preparation Time:** 10 minutes
- **Cooking Time:** 15 minutes
- **Servings:** 2

Ingredients:

- 10 large sea scallops
- 1 cup cooked millet
- 2 cups baby spinach
- 1 tbsp olive oil
- 1 tsp lemon juice

Instructions:

1. Sear scallops in olive oil 2 minutes per side.
2. Sauté spinach in same pan.
3. Serve scallops over millet with lemon drizzle.

Portion per Day: 5 scallops + spinach and millet

Nutritional Values (per serving):

- **Calories:** 340
- **Protein:** 28g
- **Carbohydrates:** 22g
- **Fats:** 16g
- **Fiber:** 5g
- **Sodium:** 120mg
- **Cholesterol:** 40mg

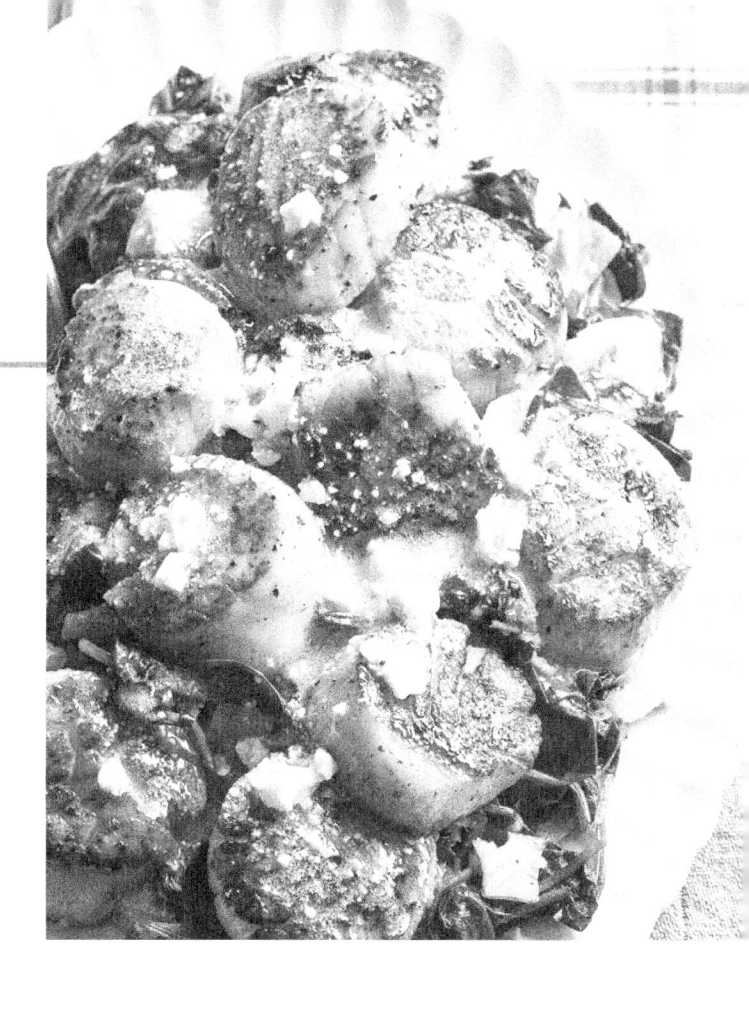

Vegetable Buckwheat Bowl with Tahini Sauce

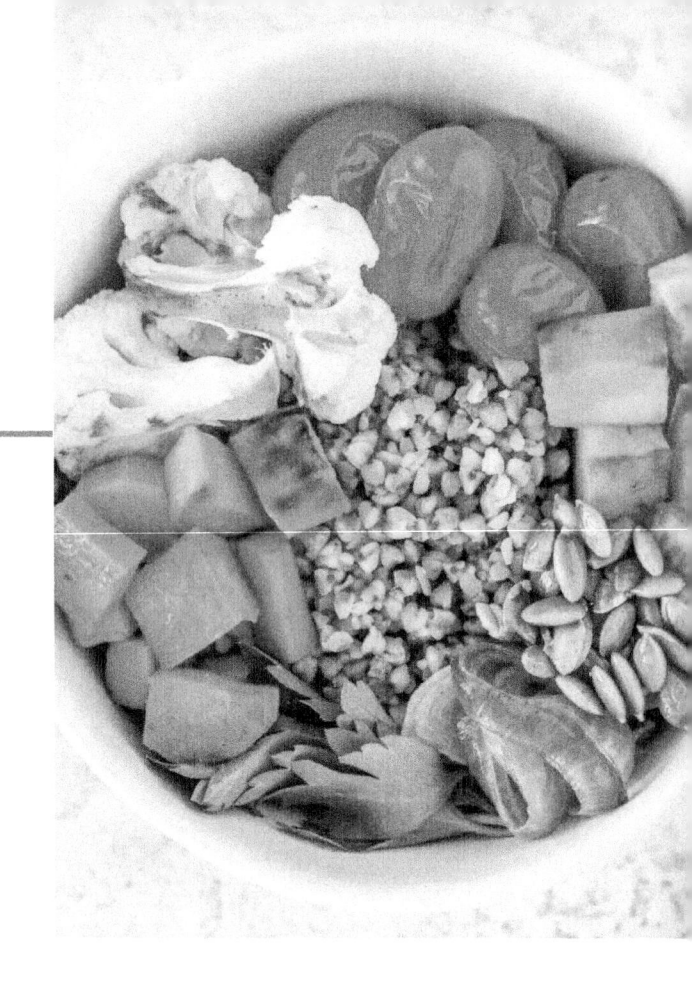

- **Preparation Time:** 10 minutes
- **Cooking Time:** 20 minutes
- **Servings:** 2

Ingredients:

- 1 cup cooked buckwheat groats
- ½ cup shredded carrots
- ½ cup steamed kale
- 1 tbsp tahini
- 1 tsp lemon juice
- 1 tsp olive oil

Instructions:

1. Mix tahini, lemon, and olive oil for dressing.
2. Combine all ingredients in a bowl and drizzle with sauce.

Portion per Day: 1 bowl

Nutritional Values (per serving):

- **Calories:** 330
- **Protein:** 15g
- **Carbohydrates:** 28g
- **Fats:** 17g
- **Fiber:** 7g
- **Sodium:** 75mg
- **Cholesterol:** 0mg

Chard and Mushroom Frittata

- **Preparation Time:** 10 minutes
- **Cooking Time:** 20 minutes
- **Servings:** 2

Ingredients:

- 4 egg whites + 2 whole eggs
- 1 cup chopped Swiss chard
- ½ cup sliced mushrooms
- 1 tbsp olive oil
- ¼ tsp black pepper

Instructions:

1. Sauté chard and mushrooms.
2. Whisk eggs and pour over vegetables.
3. Cook on low heat until set or bake at 350°F for 10–15 mins.

Portion per Day: ½ frittata

Nutritional Values (per serving):

- **Calories:** 280
- **Protein:** 22g
- **Carbohydrates:** 6g
- **Fats:** 18g
- **Fiber:** 2g
- **Sodium:** 90mg
- **Cholesterol:** 130mg

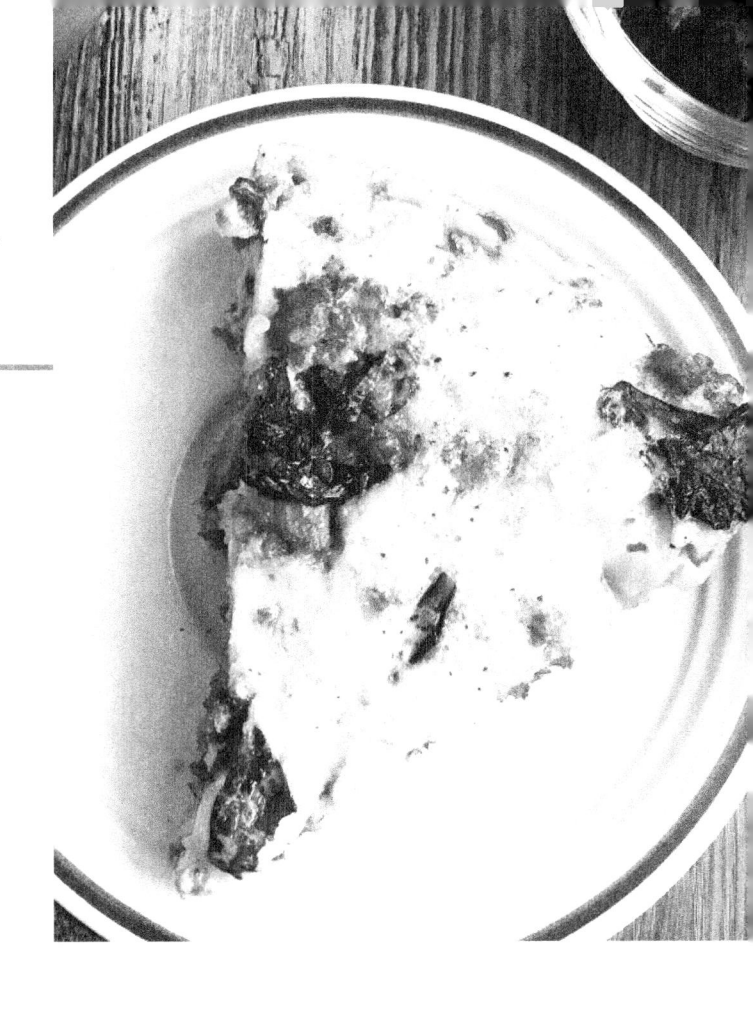

Grilled Seitan and Cabbage Slaw Wrap

- **Preparation Time:** 10 minutes
- **Cooking Time:** 10 minutes
- **Servings:** 2

Ingredients:

- 1 cup sliced seitan
- 1 cup shredded cabbage
- ½ carrot, grated
- 2 whole wheat wraps (low sodium)
- 1 tsp olive oil
- 1 tbsp lemon juice

Instructions:

1. Sauté seitan until browned.
2. Toss cabbage and carrot with lemon juice.
3. Layer slaw and seitan in wrap and roll.

Portion per Day: 1 wrap

Nutritional Values (per serving):

- **Calories:** 340
- **Protein:** 28g
- **Carbohydrates:** 22g
- **Fats:** 14g
- **Fiber:** 5g
- **Sodium:** 115mg
- **Cholesterol:** 0mg

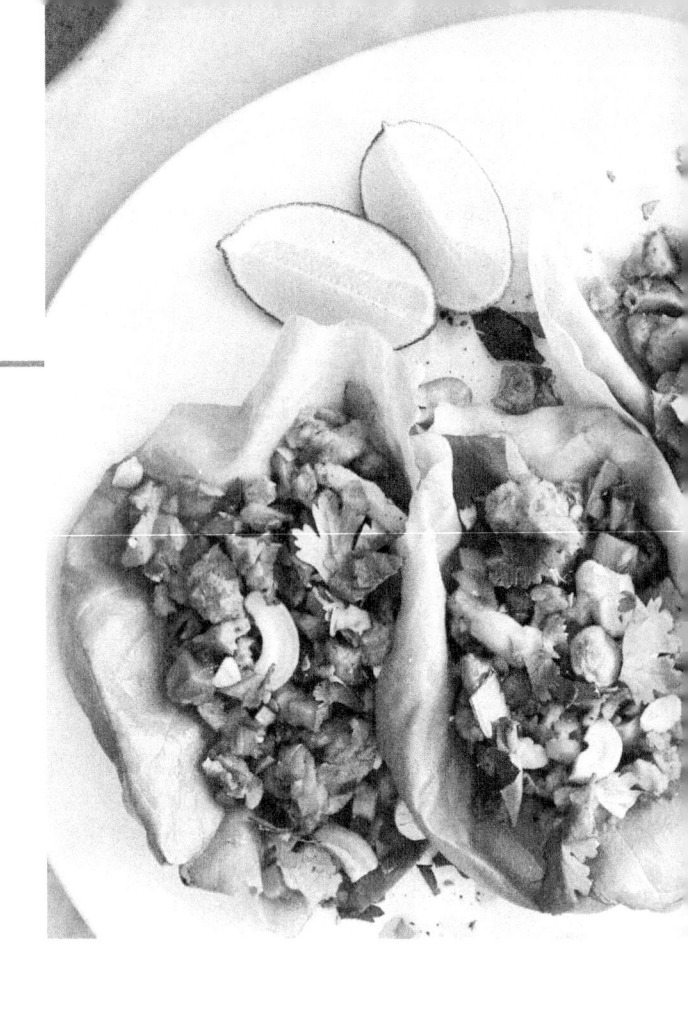

CHAPTER 07
SNACKS

Snacks often carry the stigma of being indulgent or detrimental to health, especially for individuals managing liver cirrhosis. However, with thoughtful ingredient choices and mindful preparation, it's entirely possible to enjoy sweet treats and satisfying snacks that align with liver-friendly dietary guidelines.

In this section, we've curated unique recipes that cater to cravings without compromising liver health. Each recipe is crafted to be low in saturated fats and refined sugars, moderate in carbohydrates, and free from alcohol and high-sodium ingredients. Instead, they emphasize whole foods like fruits, nuts, seeds, legumes, and natural sweeteners, providing not only delightful flavors but also nutritional benefits.

From no-bake energy bites and fruit-based desserts to wholesome muffins and savory snacks, these recipes are designed to be simple to prepare and enjoyable to consume. They offer a variety of textures and tastes, ensuring that there's something to satisfy every palate.

Whether you're seeking a midday snack, a post-meal dessert, or a healthy option to share with friends and family, this collection provides delicious choices that support liver wellness. Remember, moderation is key, and these treats are best enjoyed as part of a balanced diet.

Let's explore these liver-friendly delights that prove healthy eating can be both nourishing and indulgent.

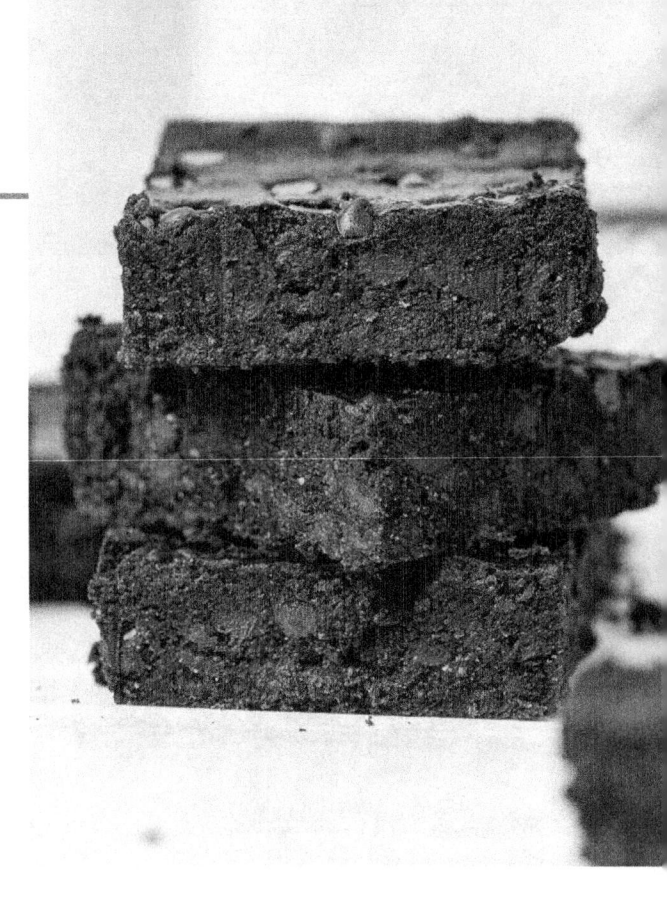

Black Bean Brownies

- **Preparation Time:** 10 minutes
- **Cooking Time:** 18 minutes
- **Servings:** 12

Ingredients:

- 1 (15 oz) can organic black beans, drained and rinsed
- 2 tablespoons cocoa powder
- 1/2 cup quick oats
- 1/4 teaspoon salt
- 1/3 cup pure maple syrup
- 1/4 cup coconut oil
- 1/2 teaspoon baking powder
- 1/2 teaspoon vanilla extract

Instructions:

1. Preheat oven to 350°F (175°C).
2. Combine all ingredients in a food processor; blend until smooth.
3. Pour batter into a greased 8x8-inch baking dish.
4. Bake for 18 minutes.
5. Allow to cool before slicing into squares.

Portion per Day: 1 brownie

Nutritional Values (per serving):

- **Calories:** 120 kcal
- **Protein:** 3 g
- **Carbohydrates:** 15 g
- **Fats:** 6 g
- **Fiber:** 3 g
- **Sodium:** 85 mg
- **Cholesterol:** 0 mg

Apple Pie Oatmeal Cookies

- **Preparation Time:** 15 minutes
- **Cooking Time:** 10 minutes
- **Servings:** 24

Ingredients:

- 1 cup rolled oats
- 1/2 cup whole wheat flour
- 1 teaspoon cinnamon
- 1/2 teaspoon baking soda
- 1/4 teaspoon salt
- 1/4 cup coconut oil, melted
- 1/4 cup honey
- 1 egg
- 1 teaspoon vanilla extract
- 1 cup finely chopped apples

Instructions:

1. Preheat oven to 350°F (175°C).
2. In a bowl, mix oats, flour, cinnamon, baking soda, and salt.
3. In another bowl, whisk coconut oil, honey, egg, and vanilla.
4. Combine wet and dry ingredients; fold in apples.
5. Drop spoonfuls onto a baking sheet; flatten slightly.
6. Bake for 10 minutes or until golden.

Portion per Day: 2 cookies

Nutritional Values (per serving):

- **Calories:** 90 kcal
- **Protein:** 2 g
- **Carbohydrates:** 14 g
- **Fats:** 3 g
- **Fiber:** 2 g
- **Sodium:** 60 mg
- **Cholesterol:** 10 mg

Roasted Chickpeas

- **Preparation Time:** 10 minutes
- **Cooking Time:** 40 minutes
- **Servings:** 4

Ingredients:

- 1 (15 oz) can chickpeas, drained and rinsed
- 1 tablespoon olive oil
- 1/2 teaspoon cumin
- 1/2 teaspoon paprika
- 1/4 teaspoon garlic powder
- Salt to taste

Instructions:

1. Preheat oven to 400°F (200°C).
2. Pat chickpeas dry; toss with olive oil and spices.
3. Spread on a baking sheet; roast for 40 minutes, shaking halfway.
4. Cool before serving.

Portion per Day: 1/2 cup

Nutritional Values (per serving):

- **Calories:** 180 kcal
- **Protein:** 7 g
- **Carbohydrates:** 20 g
- **Fats:** 8 g
- **Fiber:** 6 g
- **Sodium:** 100 mg
- **Cholesterol:** 0 mg

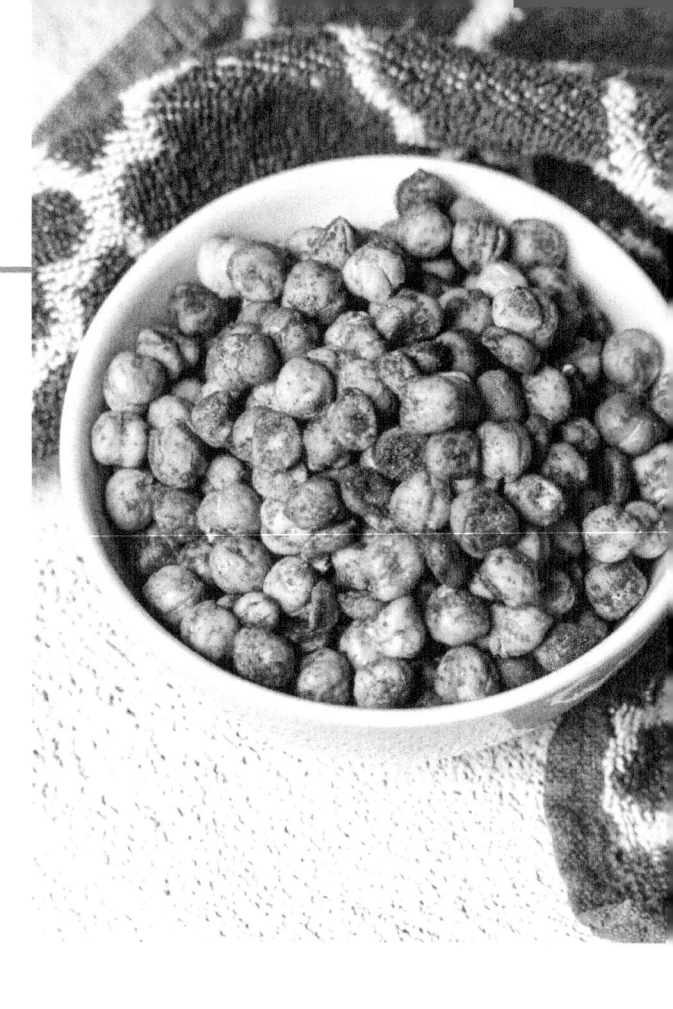

Avocado Chocolate Mousse

- **Preparation Time:** 10 minutes
- **Cooking Time:** 0 minutes
- **Servings:** 4

Ingredients:

- 2 ripe avocados
- 1/4 cup unsweetened cocoa powder
- 1/4 cup pure maple syrup
- 1/4 cup unsweetened almond milk
- 1 teaspoon vanilla extract

Instructions:

1. Scoop the flesh of the avocados into a blender or food processor.
2. Add cocoa powder, maple syrup, almond milk, and vanilla extract.
3. Blend until smooth and creamy.
4. Chill in the refrigerator for at least 30 minutes before serving.

Portion per Day: 1 serving

Nutritional Values (per serving):

- **Calories:** 180 kcal
- **Protein:** 2 g
- **Carbohydrates:** 15 g
- **Fats:** 13 g
- **Fiber:** 5 g
- **Sodium:** 10 mg
- **Cholesterol:** 0 mg

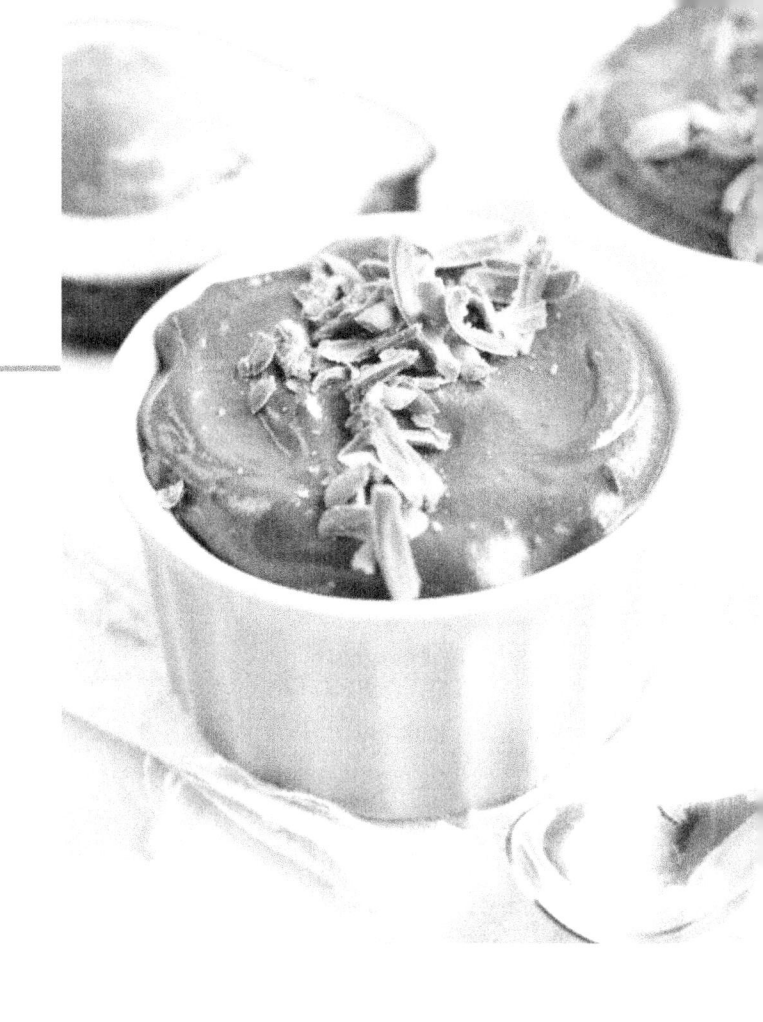

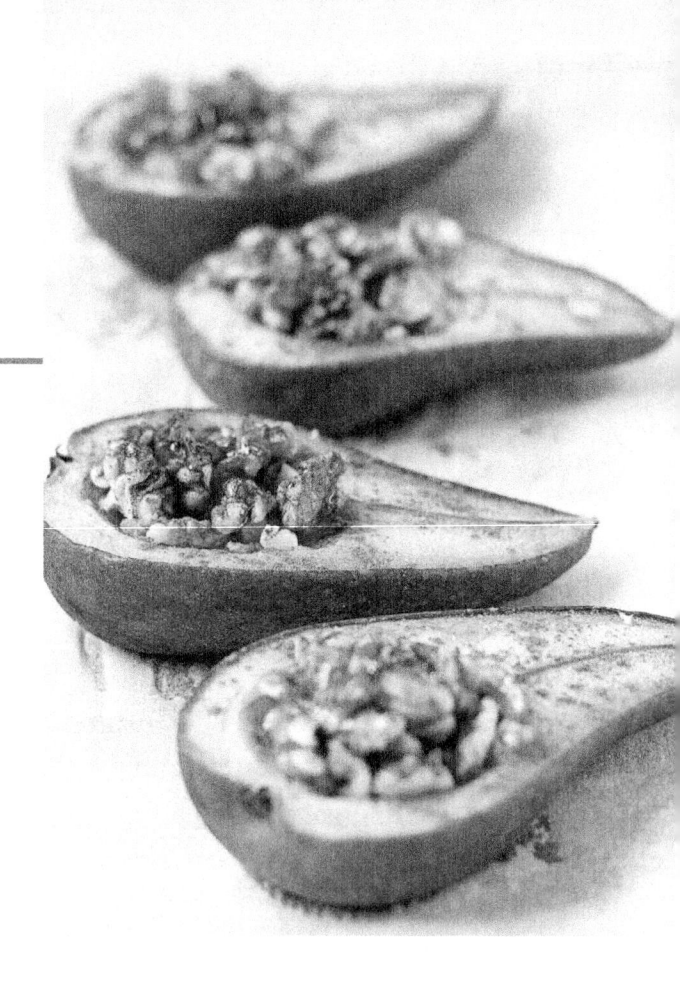

Baked Cinnamon Pears

- **Preparation Time:** 10 minutes
- **Cooking Time:** 25 minutes
- **Servings:** 2

Ingredients:

- 2 ripe pears, halved and cored
- 1 tablespoon honey
- 1/2 teaspoon ground cinnamon
- 1/4 cup chopped walnuts (optional)

Instructions:

1. Preheat oven to 350°F (175°C).
2. Place pear halves in a baking dish, cut side up.
3. Drizzle with honey and sprinkle with cinnamon.
4. Top with chopped walnuts if using.
5. Bake for 25 minutes until pears are tender.

Portion per Day: 1 pear half

Nutritional Values (per serving):

- **Calories:** 120 kcal
- **Protein:** 1 g
- **Carbohydrates:** 22 g
- **Fats:** 4 g
- **Fiber:** 4 g
- **Sodium:** 5 mg
- **Cholesterol:** 0 mg

Carrot and Oat Energy Bites

- **Preparation Time:** 15 minutes
- **Cooking Time:** 0 minutes
- **Servings:** 12

Ingredients:

- 1 cup rolled oats
- 1/2 cup grated carrots
- 1/4 cup almond butter
- 1/4 cup raisins
- 1 tablespoon honey
- 1/2 teaspoon ground cinnamon

Instructions:

1. In a bowl, mix all ingredients until well combined.
2. Roll the mixture into 1-inch balls.
3. Refrigerate for at least 30 minutes before serving.

Portion per Day: 2 energy bites

Nutritional Values (per serving):

- **Calories:** 90 kcal
- **Protein:** 2 g
- **Carbohydrates:** 12 g
- **Fats:** 4 g
- **Fiber:** 2 g
- **Sodium:** 15 mg
- **Cholesterol:** 0 mg

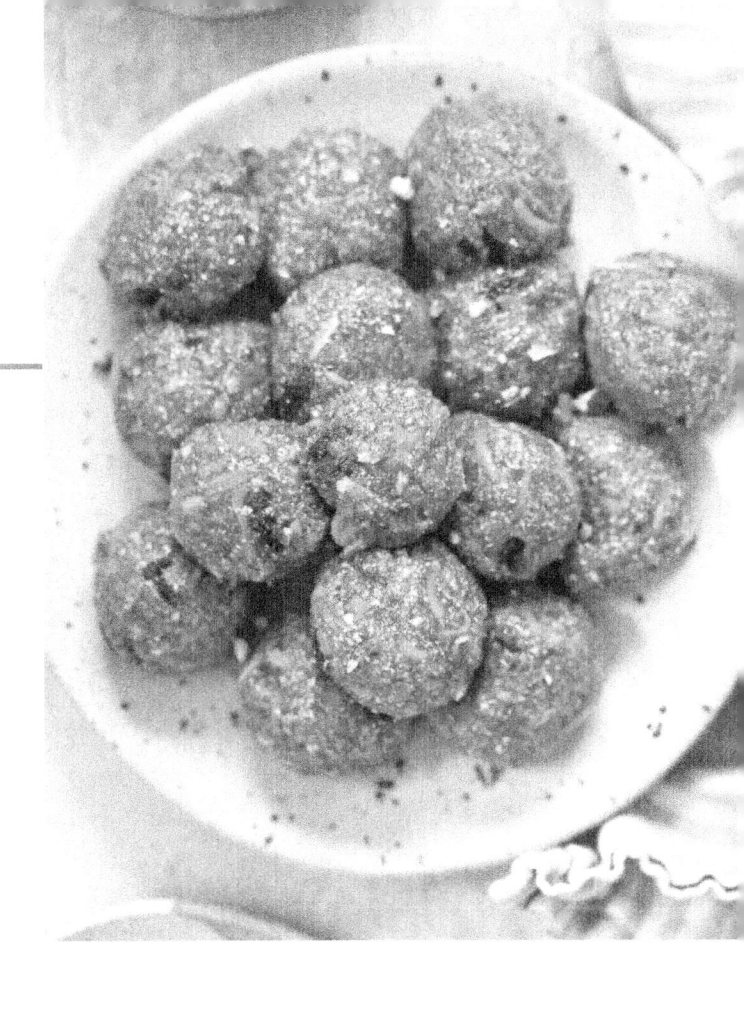

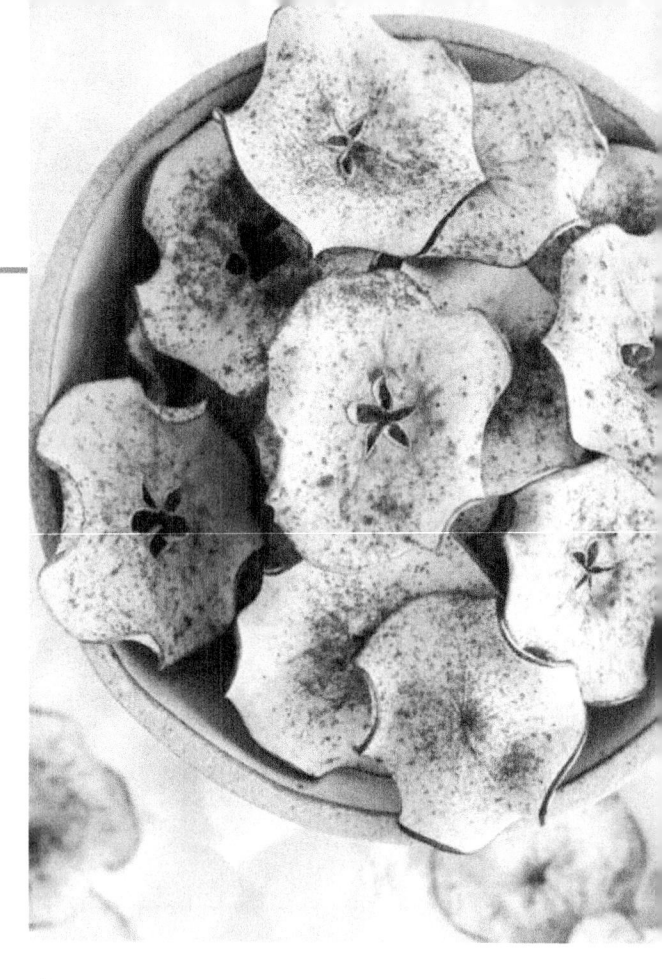

Baked Apple Chips

- **Preparation Time:** 10 minutes
- **Cooking Time:** 2 hours
- **Servings:** 4

Ingredients:

- 2 apples, thinly sliced
- 1/2 teaspoon ground cinnamon

Instructions:

1. Preheat oven to 200°F (95°C).
2. Arrange apple slices on a baking sheet lined with parchment paper.
3. Sprinkle with cinnamon.
4. Bake for 2 hours, flipping halfway through, until crisp.
5. Allow to cool before serving.

Portion per Day: 1 serving

Nutritional Values (per serving):

- **Calories:** 50 kcal
- **Protein:** 0 g
- **Carbohydrates:** 13 g
- **Fats:** 0 g
- **Fiber:** 2 g
- **Sodium:** 0 mg
- **Cholesterol:** 0 mg

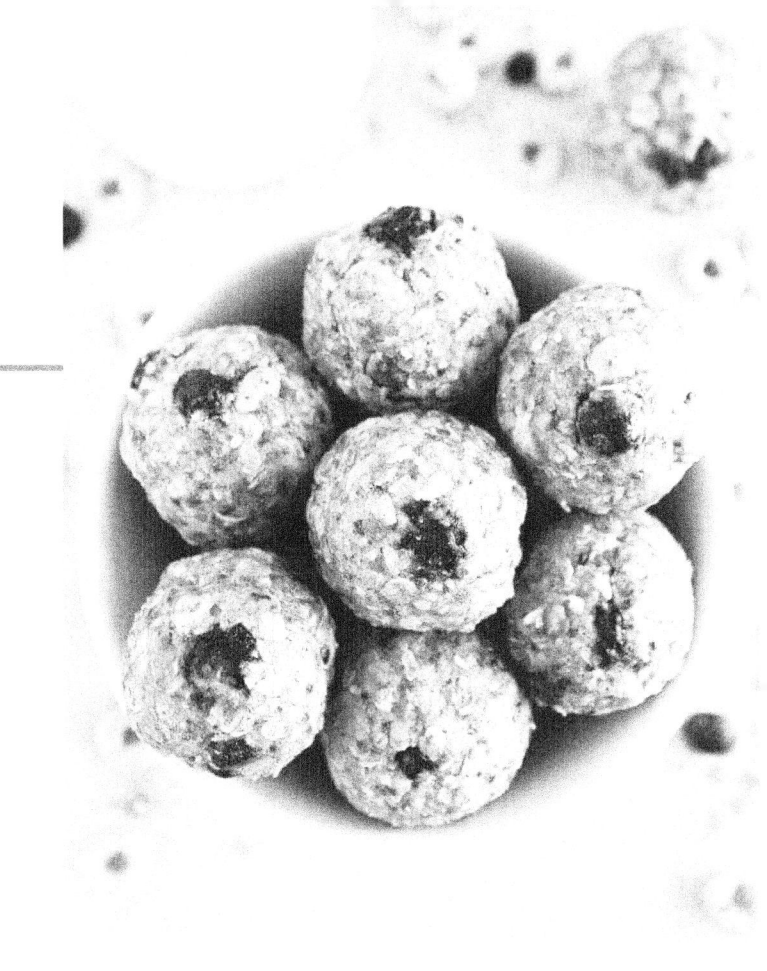

No-Bake Blueberry Energy Bites

- **Preparation Time:** 15 minutes
- **Cooking Time:** 0 minutes
- **Servings:** 12

Ingredients:

- 1 cup rolled oats
- 1/2 cup dried blueberries
- 1/4 cup almond butter
- 2 tablespoons honey
- 1/4 cup ground flaxseed
- 1/2 teaspoon vanilla extract

Instructions:

1. In a mixing bowl, combine all ingredients until well mixed.
2. Roll the mixture into 1-inch balls.
3. Place on a baking sheet and refrigerate for at least 30 minutes before serving.

Portion per Day: 2 energy bites

Nutritional Values (per serving):

- **Calories:** 100 kcal
- **Protein:** 2 g
- **Carbohydrates:** 12 g
- **Fats:** 5 g
- **Fiber:** 2 g
- **Sodium:** 10 mg
- **Cholesterol:** 0 mg

Baked Zucchini Fries

- **Preparation Time:** 10 minutes
- **Cooking Time:** 25 minutes
- **Servings:** 4

Ingredients:

- 2 medium zucchinis, cut into sticks
- 1/2 cup whole wheat breadcrumbs
- 1/4 cup grated Parmesan cheese
- 1 teaspoon dried oregano
- 1/2 teaspoon garlic powder
- 1 egg, beaten

Instructions:

1. Preheat oven to 425°F (220°C).
2. In a bowl, mix breadcrumbs, Parmesan, oregano, and garlic powder.
3. Dip zucchini sticks into the beaten egg, then coat with breadcrumb mixture.
4. Place on a baking sheet lined with parchment paper.
5. Bake for 20-25 minutes until golden and crispy.

Portion per Day: 1 serving

Nutritional Values (per serving):

- **Calories:** 110 kcal
- **Protein:** 6 g
- **Carbohydrates:** 12 g
- **Fats:** 5 g
- **Fiber:** 2 g
- **Sodium:** 150 mg
- **Cholesterol:** 40 mg

Chia & Raspberry Jam

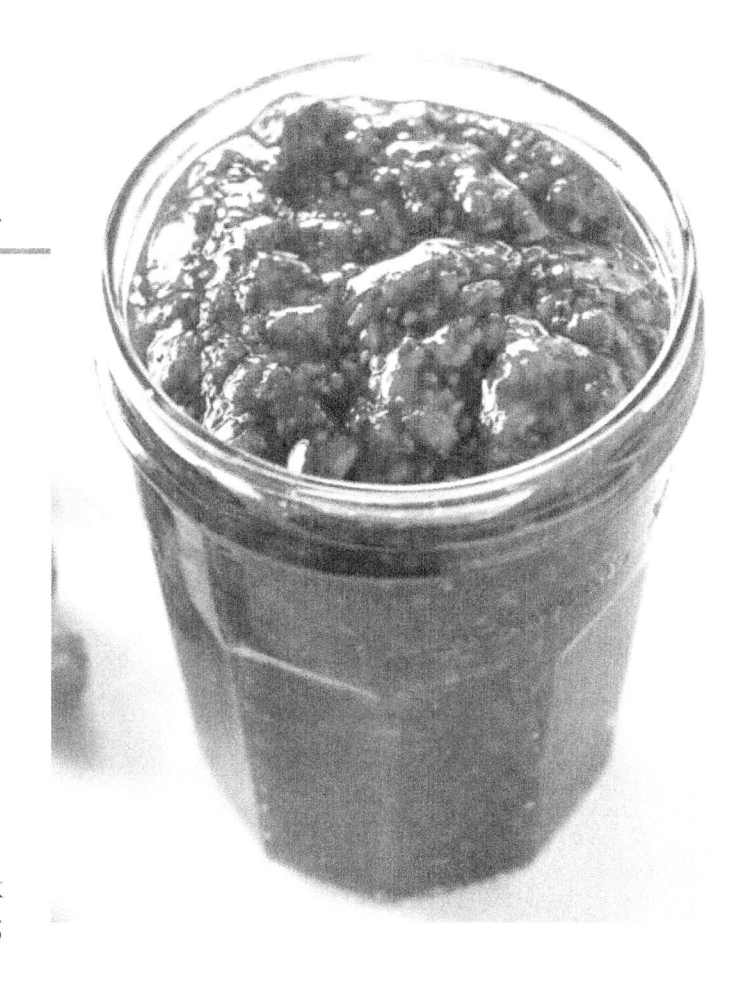

- **Preparation Time:** 5 minutes
- **Cooking Time:** 10 minutes
- **Servings:** 10

Ingredients:

- 2 cups fresh or frozen raspberries
- 2 tablespoons chia seeds
- 1 tablespoon honey
- 1/2 teaspoon vanilla extract

Instructions:

1. In a saucepan over medium heat, cook raspberries until they break down, about 5 minutes.
2. Stir in chia seeds, honey, and vanilla extract.
3. Cook for another 5 minutes, stirring frequently.
4. Remove from heat and let cool. The jam will thicken as it cools.

Portion per Day: 2 tablespoons

Nutritional Values (per serving):

- **Calories:** 30 kcal
- **Protein:** 1 g
- **Carbohydrates:** 5 g
- **Fats:** 1 g
- **Fiber:** 3 g
- **Sodium:** 0 mg
- **Cholesterol:** 0 mg

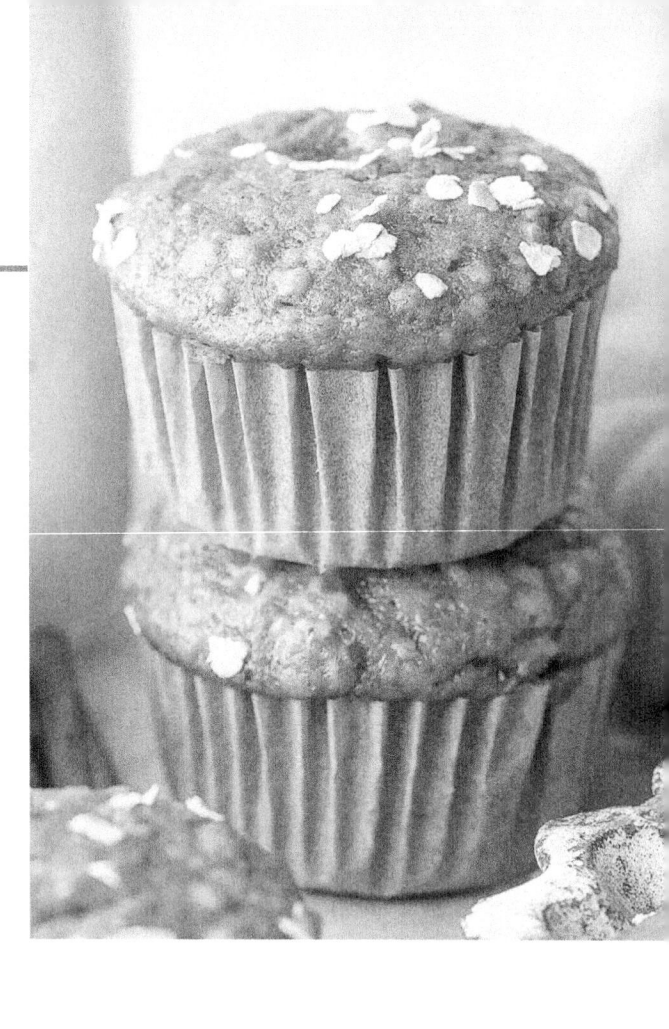

Pumpkin Oat Muffins

- **Preparation Time:** 15 minutes
- **Cooking Time:** 20 minutes
- **Servings:** 12

Ingredients:

- 1 cup canned pumpkin puree
- 2 eggs
- 1/4 cup honey
- 1/4 cup olive oil
- 1 cup whole wheat flour
- 1 cup rolled oats
- 1 teaspoon baking soda
- 1/2 teaspoon cinnamon
- 1/4 teaspoon nutmeg
- 1/4 teaspoon salt

Instructions:

1. Preheat oven to 350°F (175°C).
2. In a bowl, mix pumpkin, eggs, honey, and olive oil.
3. In another bowl, combine flour, oats, baking soda, cinnamon, nutmeg, and salt.
4. Gradually add dry ingredients to wet ingredients, mixing until just combined.
5. Divide batter into a muffin tin lined with paper cups.
6. Bake for 20 minutes or until a toothpick comes out clean.

Portion per Day: 1 muffin

Nutritional Values (per serving):

- **Calories:** 150 kcal
- **Protein:** 3 g
- **Carbohydrates:** 20 g
- **Fats:** 6 g
- **Fiber:** 3 g
- **Sodium:** 120 mg
- **Cholesterol:** 35 mg

Baked Sweet Potato Chips

- **Preparation Time:** 10 minutes
- **Cooking Time:** 30 minutes
- **Servings:** 4

Ingredients:

- 2 medium sweet potatoes, thinly sliced
- 1 tablespoon olive oil
- 1/2 teaspoon paprika
- 1/4 teaspoon sea salt

Instructions:

1. Preheat oven to 400°F (200°C).
2. Toss sweet potato slices with olive oil, paprika, and sea salt.
3. Arrange on a baking sheet in a single layer.
4. Bake for 25-30 minutes, flipping halfway through, until crispy.

Portion per Day: 1 serving

Nutritional Values (per serving):

- **Calories:** 120 kcal
- **Protein:** 2 g
- **Carbohydrates:** 20 g
- **Fats:** 4 g
- **Fiber:** 3 g
- **Sodium:** 100 mg
- **Cholesterol:** 0 mg

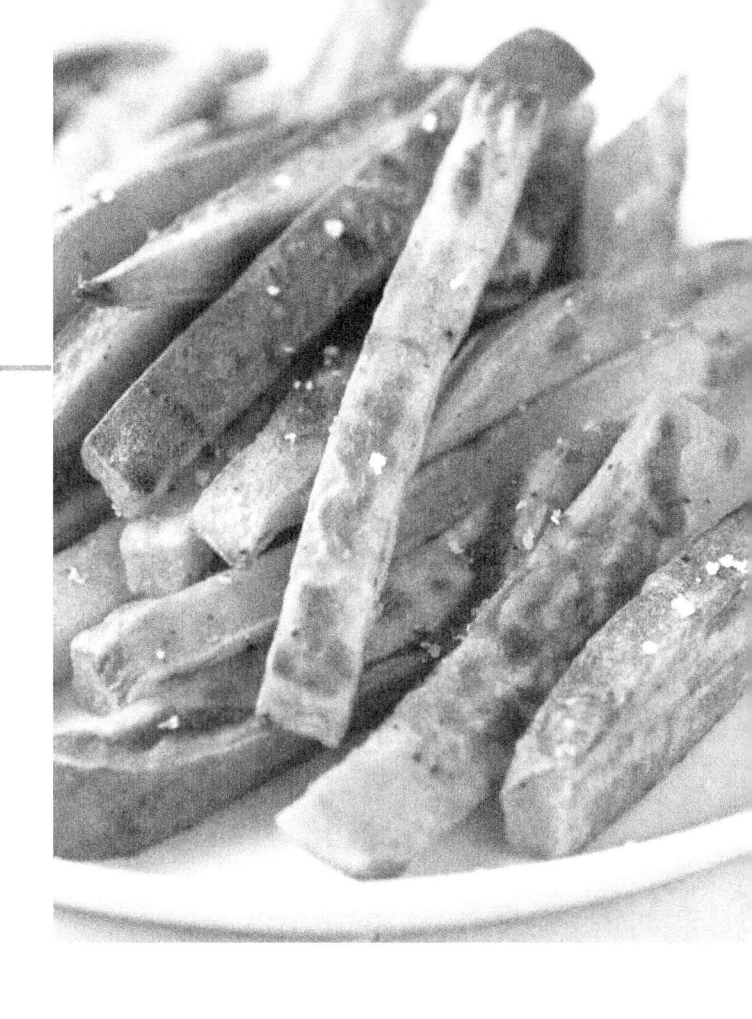

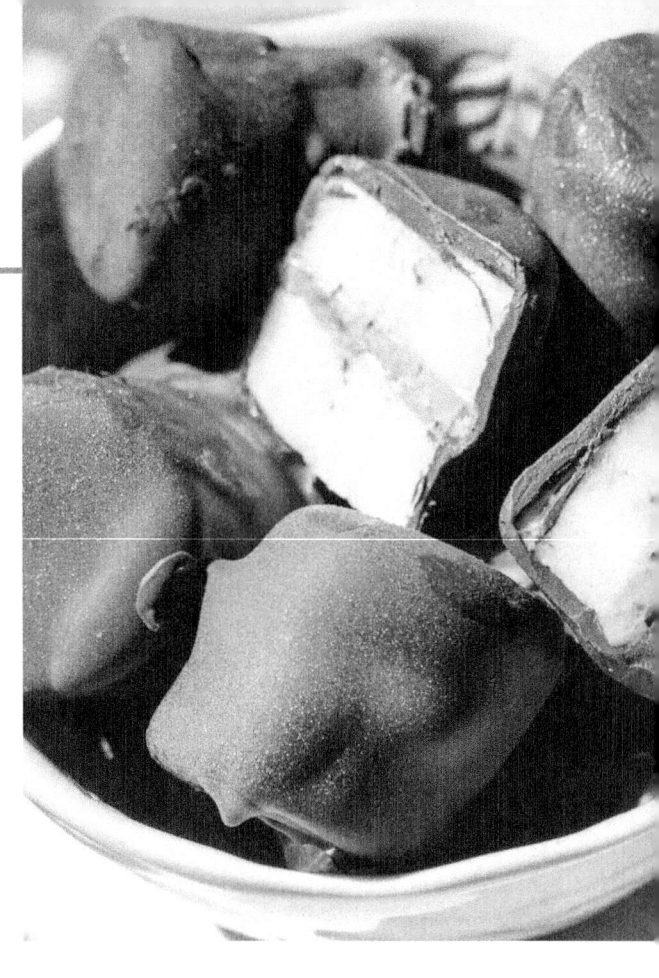

Frozen Banana Bites

- **Preparation Time:** 15 minutes (plus freezing time)
- **Cooking Time:** 0 minutes
- **Servings:** 6

Ingredients:

- 2 ripe bananas, sliced
- 1/4 cup dark chocolate chips (70% cocoa)
- 1 tablespoon chopped nuts (optional)

Instructions:

1. Place banana slices on a baking sheet lined with parchment paper.
2. Melt dark chocolate chips in a microwave-safe bowl.
3. Dip banana slices halfway into melted chocolate and place back on the baking sheet.
4. Sprinkle with chopped nuts if desired.
5. Freeze for at least 2 hours before serving.

Portion per Day: 2-3 banana bites

Nutritional Values (per serving):

- **Calories:** 90 kcal
- **Protein:** 1 g
- **Carbohydrates:** 15 g
- **Fats:** 3 g
- **Fiber:** 2 g
- **Sodium:** 0 mg
- **Cholesterol:** 0 mg

CHAPTER 08

DRINKS

Hydration is vital for liver cirrhosis management, especially for seniors with reduced appetites. Beverages can deliver essential nutrients without overwhelming digestion, but commercial options often contain sugars, sodium, and additives that burden an already compromised liver.

This collection features therapeutic smoothies and drinks specifically formulated to support liver health. Each recipe delivers targeted benefits through antioxidant-rich, anti-inflammatory ingredients like berries, leafy greens, citrus, cucumber, ginger, and turmeric. These aren't merely fruit blends—they're functional beverages addressing specific health needs.

You won't find refined sugars, alcohol, high-fat dairy, or excessive sodium here. Instead, these balanced options range from energizing to calming, with varieties including creamy smoothies, herbal teas, fruit-vegetable juices, infused waters, and healing tonics. Each serves a purpose: reducing inflammation, aiding digestion, stabilizing blood sugar, or providing refreshment.

Simple to prepare and gentle on digestion, these drinks can be enjoyed throughout the day, helping maintain consistent nutrition even when eating is difficult. Every sip works subtly to improve liver function and enhance overall well-being.

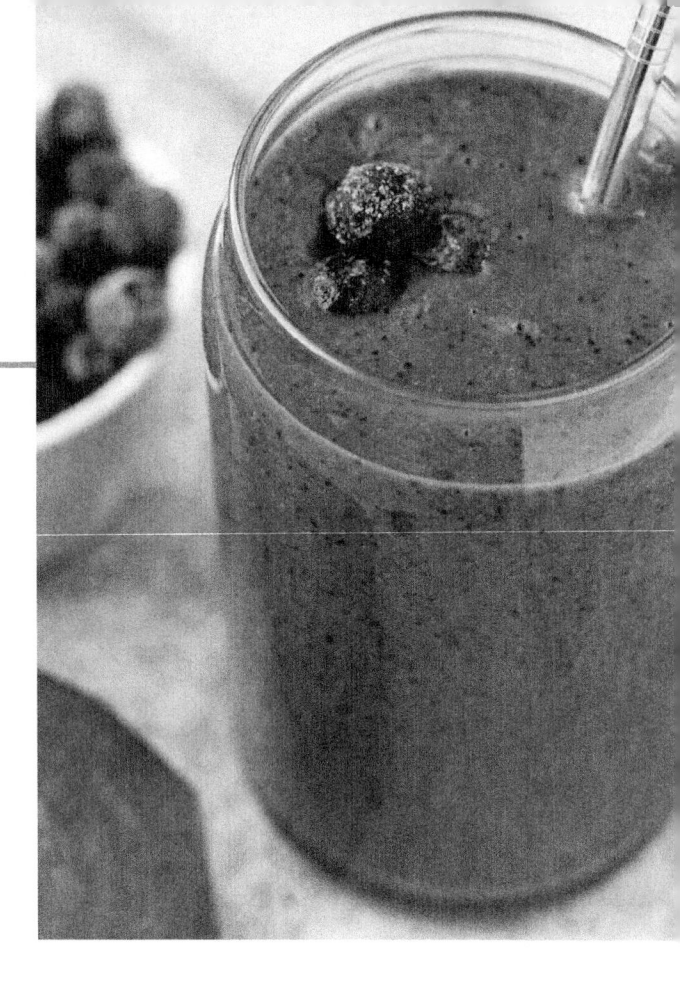

Beetroot & Berry Detox Smoothie

- **Preparation Time:** 10 minutes
- **Cooking Time:** 0 minutes
- **Servings:** 2

Ingredients:

- 1 medium beetroot, peeled and chopped
- 1 cup frozen mixed berries
- 1/2 cup unsweetened almond milk
- 1 tablespoon chia seeds
- 1 teaspoon honey (optional)

Instructions:

1. Blend all ingredients until smooth.
2. Serve immediately.

Portion per Day: 1 serving

Nutritional Values (per serving):

- **Calories:** 120 kcal
- **Protein:** 3 g
- **Carbohydrates:** 25 g
- **Fats:** 2 g
- **Fiber:** 6 g
- **Sodium:** 50 mg
- **Cholesterol:** 0 mg

Green Tea & Citrus Refresher

- **Preparation Time:** 5 minutes (plus cooling time)
- **Cooking Time:** 0 minutes
- **Servings:** 2

Ingredients:

- 2 cups brewed green tea, cooled
- 1/2 cup fresh orange juice
- 1 tablespoon lemon juice
- 1 teaspoon grated ginger
- Ice cubes

Instructions:

1. Combine all ingredients in a pitcher.
2. Serve over ice.

Portion per Day: 1 serving

Nutritional Values (per serving):

- **Calories:** 60 kcal
- **Protein:** 0 g
- **Carbohydrates:** 15 g
- **Fats:** 0 g
- **Fiber:** 0 g
- **Sodium:** 5 mg
- **Cholesterol:** 0 mg

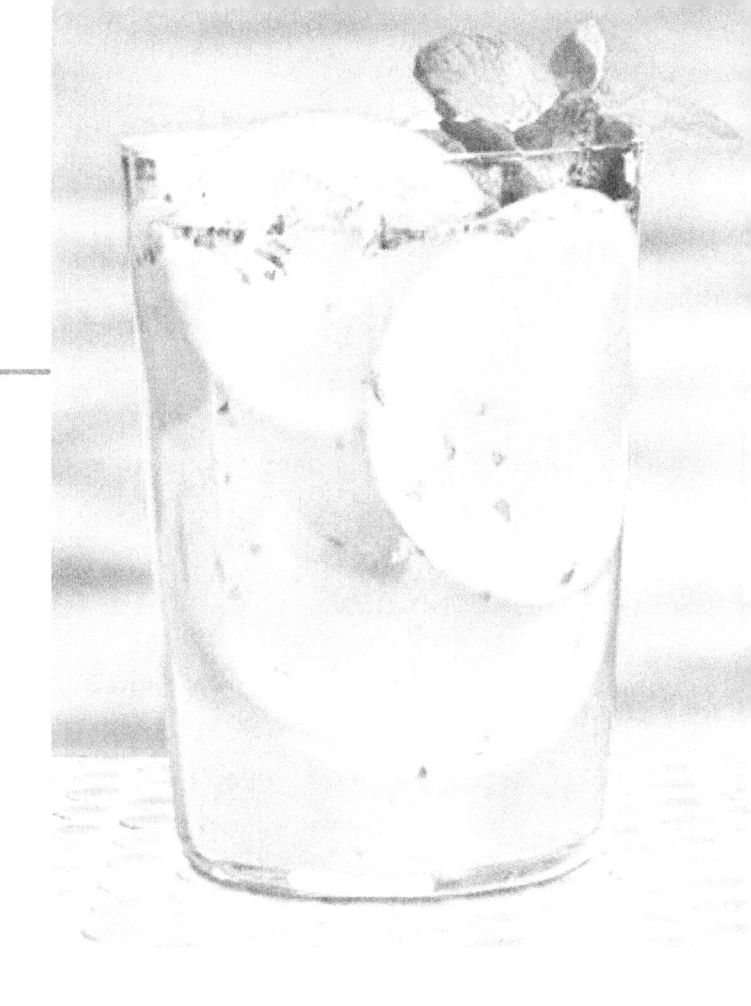

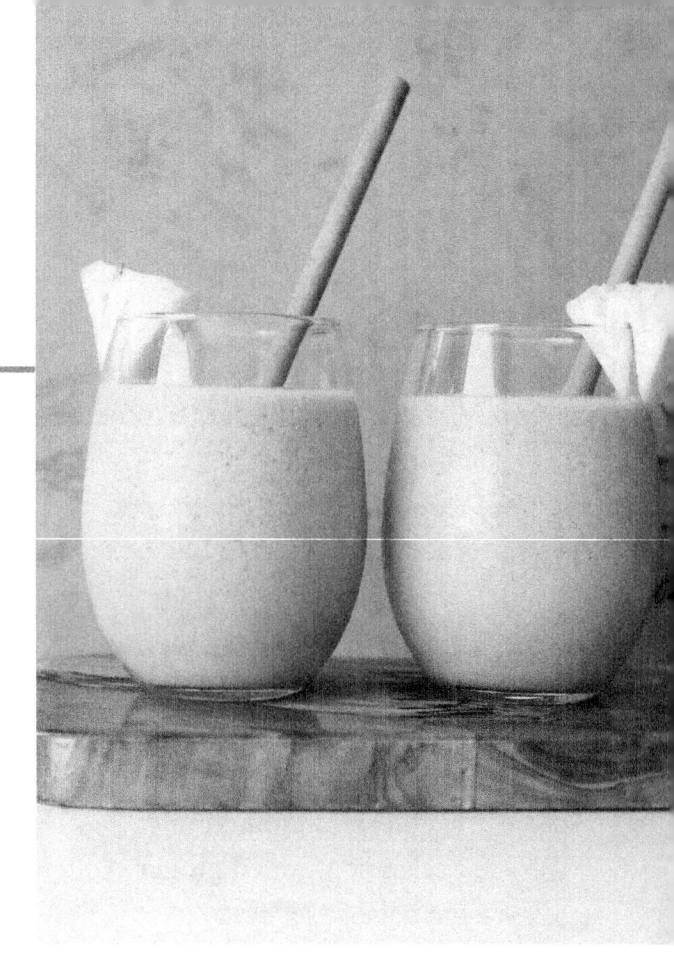

Turmeric & Pineapple Smoothie

- **Preparation Time:** 10 minutes
- **Cooking Time:** 0 minutes
- **Servings:** 2

Ingredients:

- 1 cup fresh pineapple chunks
- 1 banana
- 1/2 teaspoon ground turmeric
- 1/2 cup unsweetened coconut water
- 1 tablespoon flaxseeds

Instructions:

1. Blend all ingredients until smooth.
2. Serve immediately.

Portion per Day: 1 serving

Nutritional Values (per serving):

- **Calories:** 140 kcal
- **Protein:** 2 g
- **Carbohydrates:** 30 g
- **Fats:** 3 g
- **Fiber:** 4 g
- **Sodium:** 10 mg
- **Cholesterol:** 0 mg

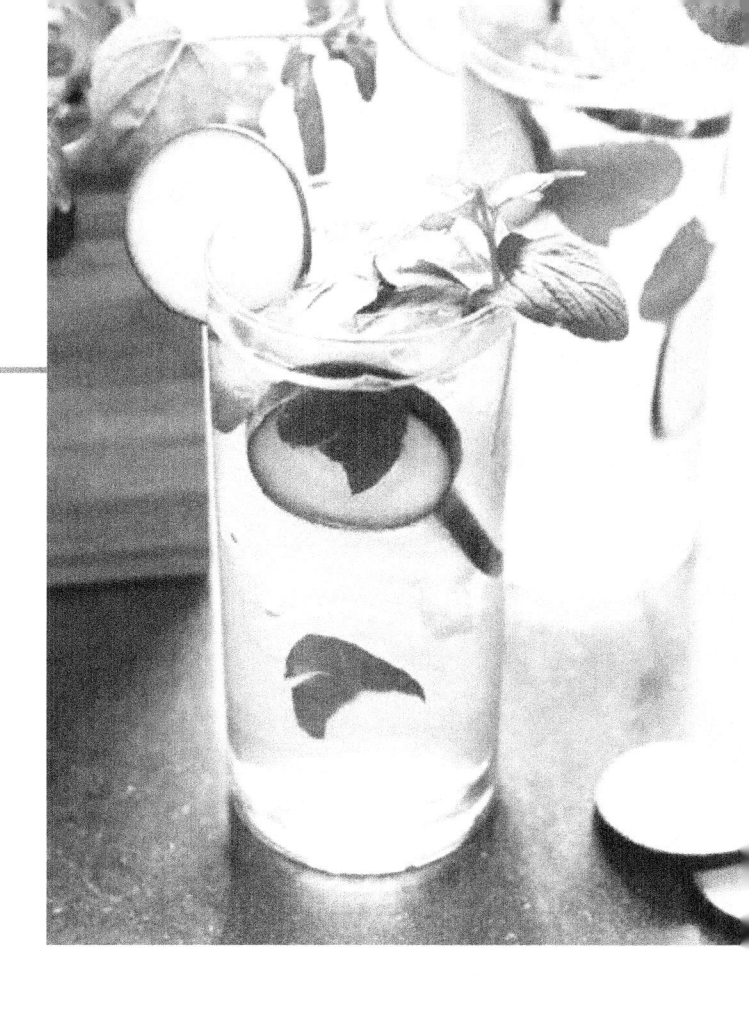

Cucumber & Mint Cooler

- **Preparation Time:** 5 minutes
- **Cooking Time:** 0 minutes
- **Servings:** 2

Ingredients:

- 1 cucumber, peeled and sliced
- 1/4 cup fresh mint leaves
- 1 tablespoon lemon juice
- 1 teaspoon honey (optional)
- 2 cups cold water

Instructions:

1. Blend all ingredients until smooth.
2. Strain and serve over ice.

Portion per Day: 1 serving

Nutritional Values (per serving):

- **Calories:** 40 kcal
- **Protein:** 1 g
- **Carbohydrates:** 10 g
- **Fats:** 0 g
- **Fiber:** 1 g
- **Sodium:** 5 mg
- **Cholesterol:** 0 mg

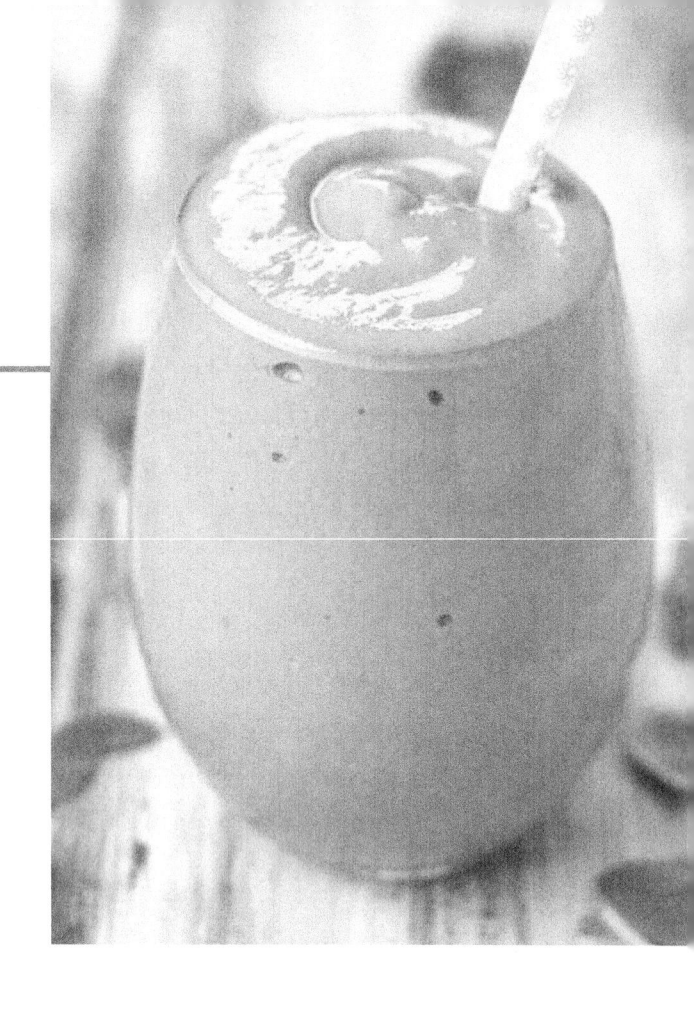

Avocado & Spinach Smoothie

- **Preparation Time:** 10 minutes
- **Cooking Time:** 0 minutes
- **Servings:** 2

Ingredients:

- 1/2 avocado
- 1 cup fresh spinach
- 1/2 cup unsweetened almond milk
- 1/2 banana
- 1 tablespoon hemp seeds

Instructions:

1. Blend all ingredients until smooth.
2. Serve immediately.

Portion per Day: 1 serving

Nutritional Values (per serving):

- **Calories:** 180 kcal
- **Protein:** 4 g
- **Carbohydrates:** 15 g
- **Fats:** 12 g
- **Fiber:** 5 g
- **Sodium:** 30 mg
- **Cholesterol:** 0 mg

Carrot-Apple Detox Juice

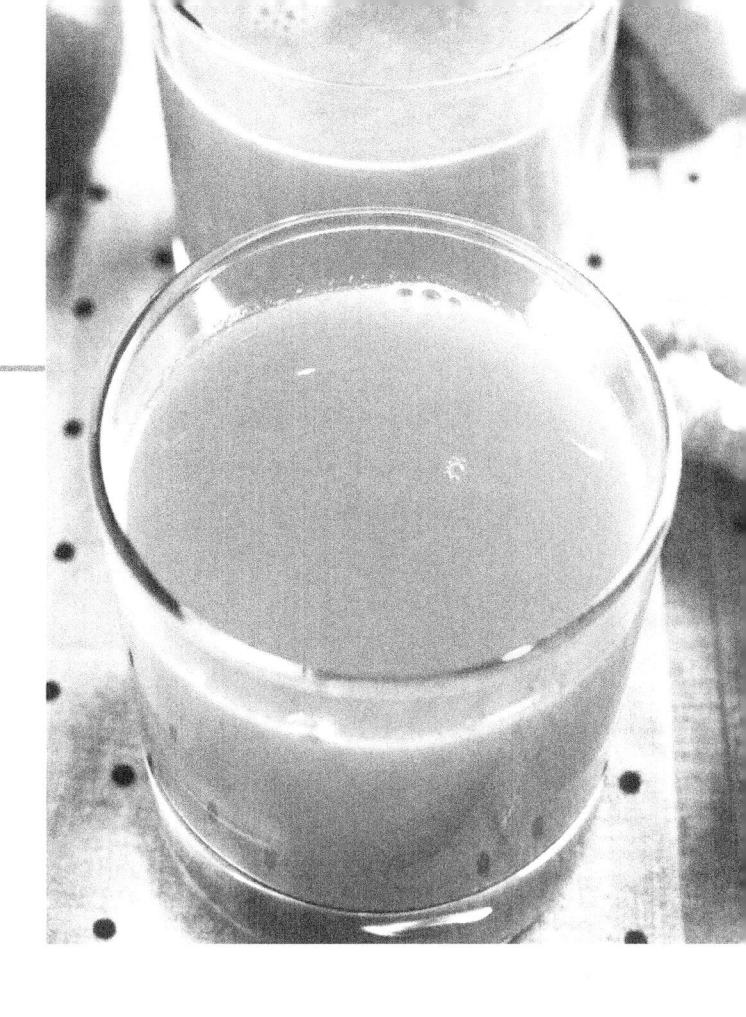

- **Preparation Time:** 10 minutes
- **Cooking Time:** 0 minutes
- **Servings:**

Ingredients:

- 2 medium carrots, peeled and chopped
- 1 apple, cored and chopped
- 1/2 inch piece of fresh turmeric root (or 1/2 teaspoon ground turmeric)
- 1 tablespoon lemon juice
- 1 cup cold water

Instructions:

1. Place all ingredients in a blender.
2. Blend until smooth.
3. Strain through a fine mesh sieve or cheesecloth if desired.
4. Serve chilled.

Portion per Day: 1 serving

Nutritional Values (per serving):

- **Calories:** 80 kcal
- **Protein:** 1 g
- **Carbohydrates:** 18 g
- **Fats:** 0.5 g
- **Fiber:** 3 g
- **Sodium:** 25 mg
- **Cholesterol:** 0 mg

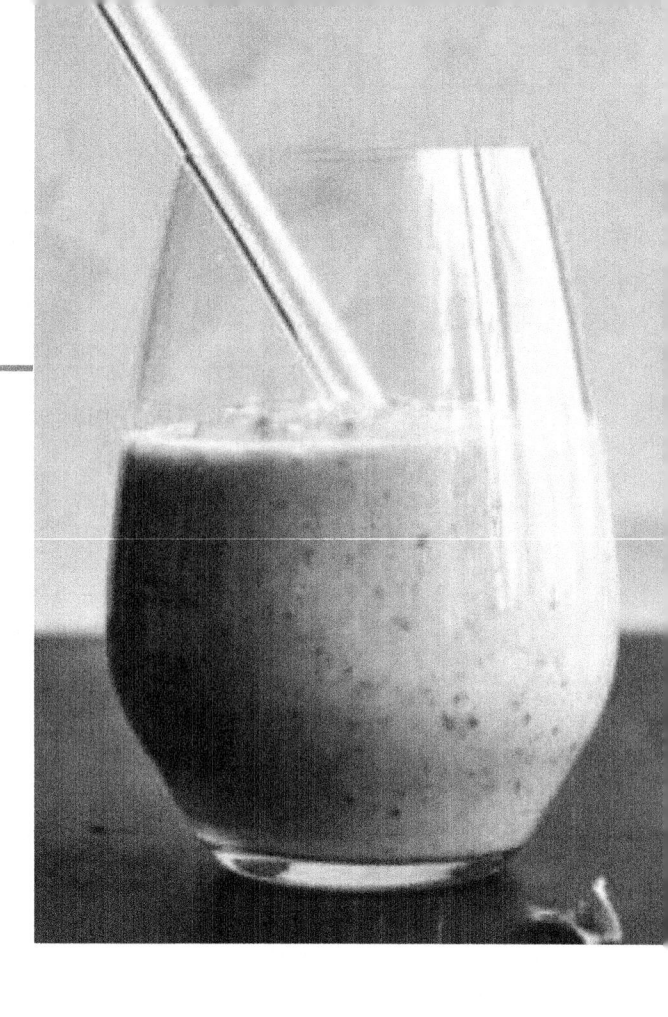

Avocado-Cilantro Smoothie

- **Preparation Time:** 10 minutes
- **Cooking Time:** 0 minutes
- **Servings:** 2

Ingredients:

- 1/2 ripe avocado
- 1/4 cup fresh cilantro leaves
- 1/2 cup pineapple chunks (fresh or frozen)
- 1 tablespoon lime juice
- 1 cup unsweetened almond milk
- Ice cubes (optional)

Instructions:

1. Combine all ingredients in a blender.
2. Blend until creamy and smooth.
3. Add ice cubes if desired and blend again.
4. Serve immediately.

Portion per Day: 1 serving

Nutritional Values (per serving):

- **Calories:** 160 kcal
- **Protein:** 2 g
- **Carbohydrates:** 10 g
- **Fats:** 13 g
- **Fiber:** 5 g
- **Sodium:** 40 mg
- **Cholesterol:** 0 mg

Berry-Lemon Infused Water

- **Preparation Time:** 5 minutes (plus infusion time)
- **Cooking Time:** 0 minutes
- **Servings:** 4

Ingredients:

- 1/2 cup mixed berries (strawberries, blueberries, raspberries)
- 1 lemon, thinly sliced
- 1 quart cold water
- Fresh mint leaves (optional)

Instructions:

1. Place berries, lemon slices, and mint leaves into a pitcher.
2. Fill with cold water.
3. Refrigerate for at least 2 hours to allow flavors to infuse.
4. Serve chilled.

Portion per Day: 1-2 servings

Nutritional Values (per serving):

- **Calories:** 10 kcal
- **Protein:** 0 g
- **Carbohydrates:** 2 g
- **Fats:** 0 g
- **Fiber:** 0.5 g
- **Sodium:** 0 mg
- **Cholesterol:** 0 mg

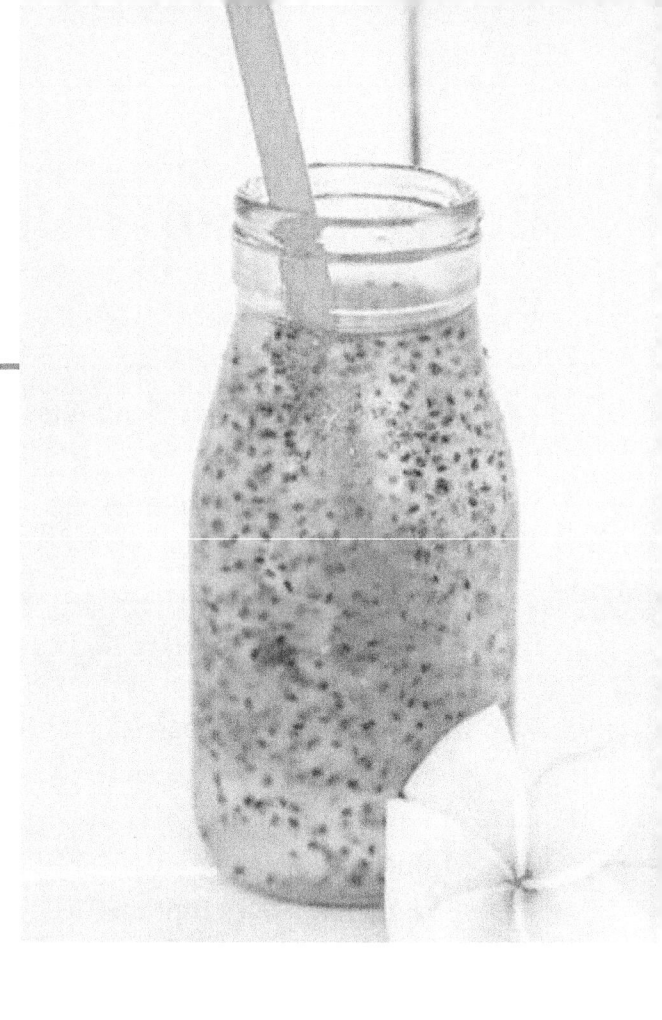

Coconut Water & Chia Refresher

- **Preparation Time:** 5 minutes (plus soaking time)
- **Cooking Time:** 0 minutes
- **Servings:** 2

Ingredients:

- 2 cups unsweetened coconut water
- 1 tablespoon chia seeds
- 1 tablespoon fresh lime juice
- 1 teaspoon honey (optional)

Instructions:

1. In a pitcher, combine coconut water, chia seeds, lime juice, and honey.
2. Stir well and let sit for at least 30 minutes to allow chia seeds to swell.
3. Stir again before serving.
4. Serve chilled.

Portion per Day: 1 serving

Nutritional Values (per serving):

- **Calories:** 60 kcal
- **Protein:** 1 g
- **Carbohydrates:** 8 g
- **Fats:** 3 g
- **Fiber:** 4 g
- **Sodium:** 40 mg
- **Cholesterol:** 0 mg

Apple-Celery Liver Cleanser

- **Preparation Time:** 10 minutes
- **Cooking Time:** 0 minutes
- **Servings:** 2

Ingredients:

- 2 green apples, cored and chopped
- 2 celery stalks, chopped
- 1 cup fresh spinach leaves
- 1 tablespoon fresh lemon juice
- 1 cup cold water

Instructions:

1. Combine all ingredients in a blender.
2. Blend until smooth.
3. Serve immediately over ice if desired.

Portion per Day: 1 serving

Nutritional Values (per serving):

- **Calories:** 90 kcal
- **Protein:** 2 g
- **Carbohydrates:** 22 g
- **Fats:** 0.5 g
- **Fiber:** 4 g
- **Sodium:** 30 mg
- **Cholesterol:** 0 mg

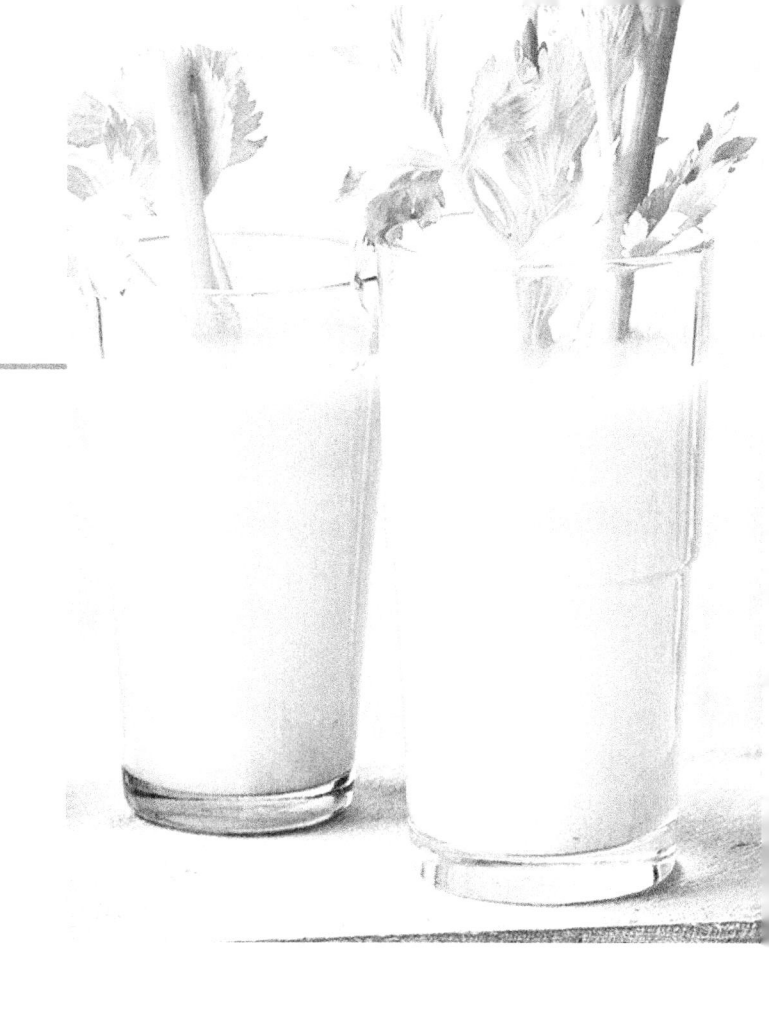

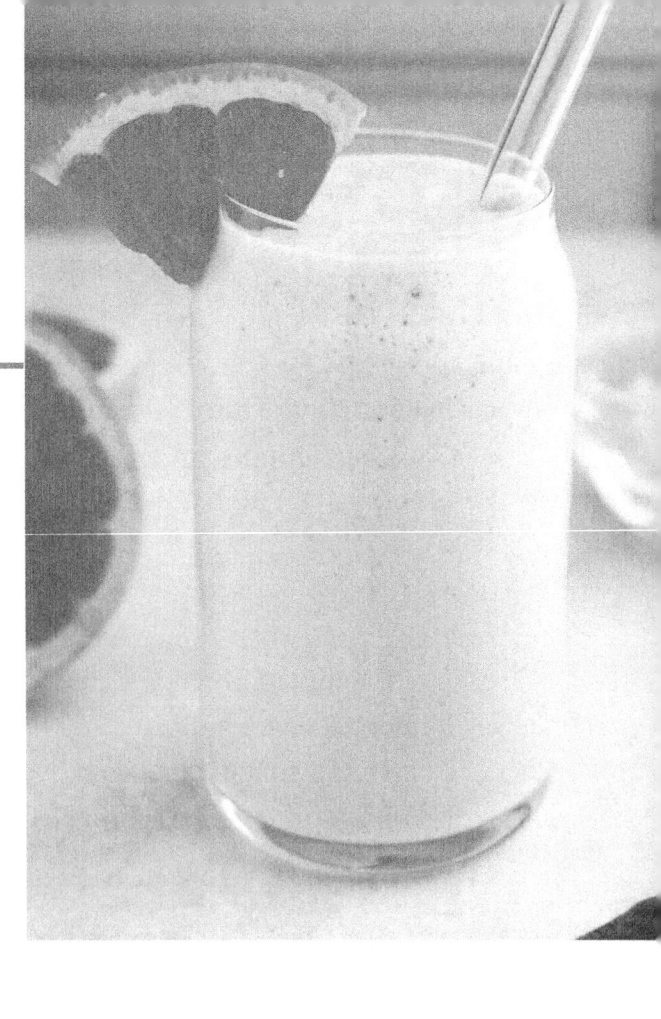

Grapefruit & Kefir Smoothie

- **Preparation Time:** 10 minutes
- **Cooking Time:** 0 minutes
- **Servings:** 2

Ingredients:

- 1 pink grapefruit, peeled and segmented
- 1/2 cup plain kefir
- 1/2 cup Greek yogurt
- 1 tablespoon honey (optional)
- 1/2 cup ice cubes

Instructions:

1. Place all ingredients in a blender.
2. Blend until smooth and creamy.
3. Serve immediately.

Portion per Day: 1 serving

Nutritional Values (per serving):

- **Calories:** 150 kcal
- **Protein:** 6 g
- **Carbohydrates:** 20 g
- **Fats:** 4 g
- **Fiber:** 2 g
- **Sodium:** 50 mg
- **Cholesterol:** 10 mg

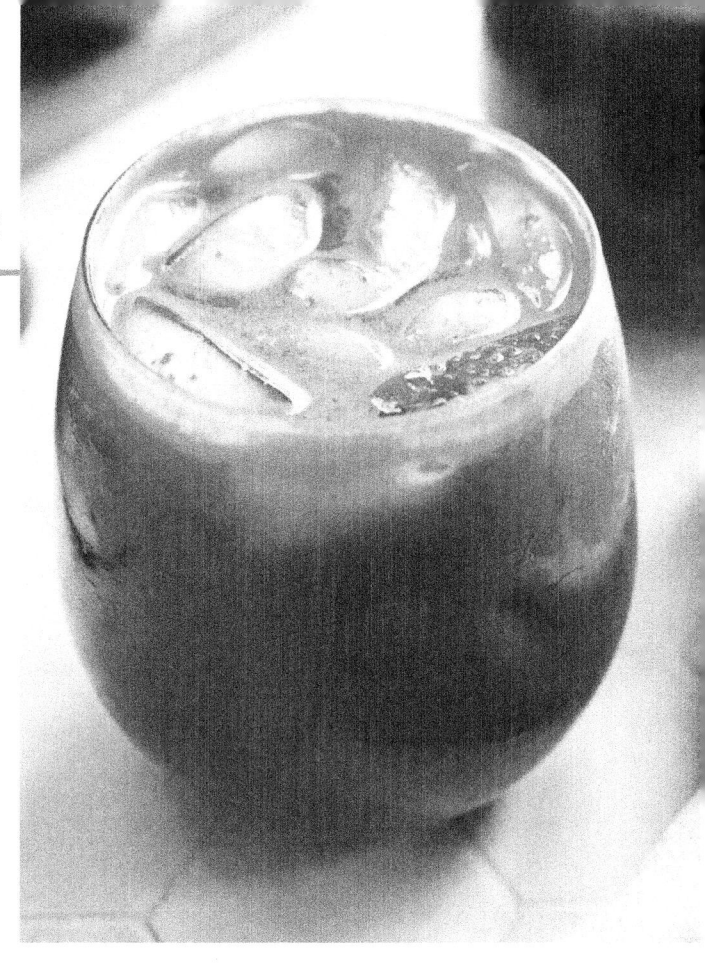

Beetroot & Carrot Juice

- **Preparation Time:** 15 minutes
- **Cooking Time:** 0 minutes
- **Servings:** 2

Ingredients:

- 1 medium beetroot, peeled and chopped
- 2 medium carrots, peeled and chopped
- 1 apple, cored and chopped
- 1 tablespoon fresh lemon juice
- 1 cup cold water

Instructions:

1. Combine all ingredients in a blender.
2. Blend until smooth.
3. Strain through a fine mesh sieve if desired.
4. Serve chilled.

Portion per Day: 1 serving

Nutritional Values (per serving):

- **Calories:** 110 kcal
- **Protein:** 2 g
- **Carbohydrates:** 25 g
- **Fats:** 0.5 g
- **Fiber:** 5 g
- **Sodium:** 40 mg
- **Cholesterol:** 0 mg

Turmeric & Ginger Tea

- **Preparation Time:** 5 minutes (plus steeping time)
- **Cooking Time:** 0 minutes
- **Servings:** 2

Ingredients:

- 2 cups hot water
- 1 teaspoon ground turmeric
- 1 teaspoon grated fresh ginger
- 1 tablespoon lemon juice
- 1 teaspoon honey (optional)

Instructions:

1. In a teapot or heatproof container, combine all ingredients.
2. Let steep for 10 minutes.
3. Strain if desired and serve warm.

Portion per Day: 1 cup

Nutritional Values (per serving):

- **Calories:** 25 kcal
- **Protein:** 0 g
- **Carbohydrates:** 6 g
- **Fats:** 0 g
- **Fiber:** 0.5 g
- **Sodium:** 5 mg
- **Cholesterol:** 0 mg

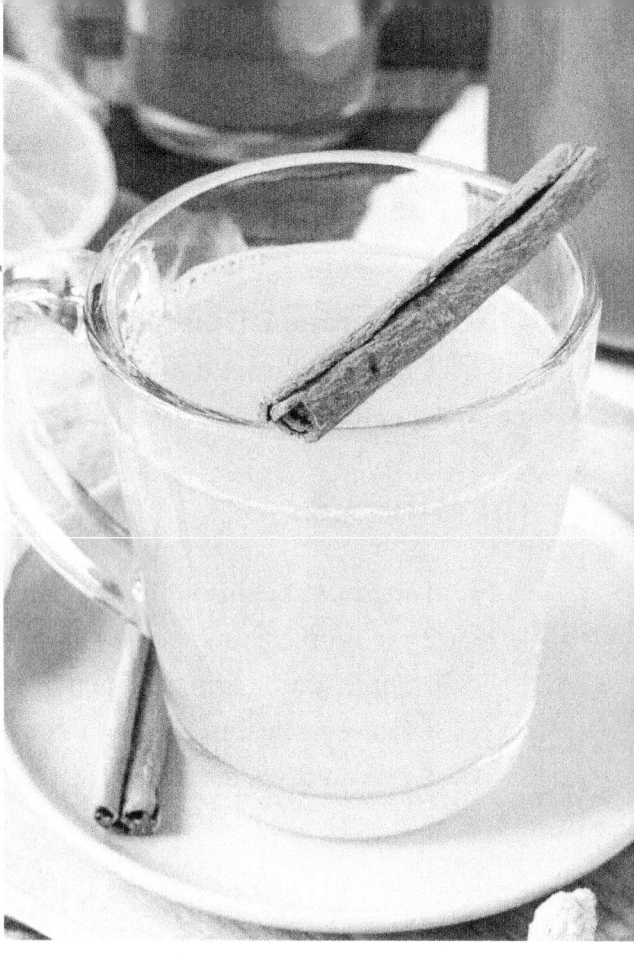

Blueberry & Avocado Smoothie

- **Preparation Time:** 10 minutes
- **Cooking Time:** 0 minutes
- **Servings:** 2

Ingredients:

- 1 cup fresh or frozen blueberries
- 1/2 ripe avocado
- 1 cup unsweetened almond milk
- 1 tablespoon chia seeds
- 1 teaspoon honey (optional)

Instructions:

1. Combine all ingredients in a blender.
2. Blend until smooth and creamy.
3. Serve immediately.

Portion per Day: 1 serving

Nutritional Values (per serving):

- **Calories:** 180 kcal
- **Protein:** 3 g
- **Carbohydrates:** 20 g
- **Fats:** 10 g
- **Fiber:** 6 g
- **Sodium:** 30 mg
- **Cholesterol:** 0 mg

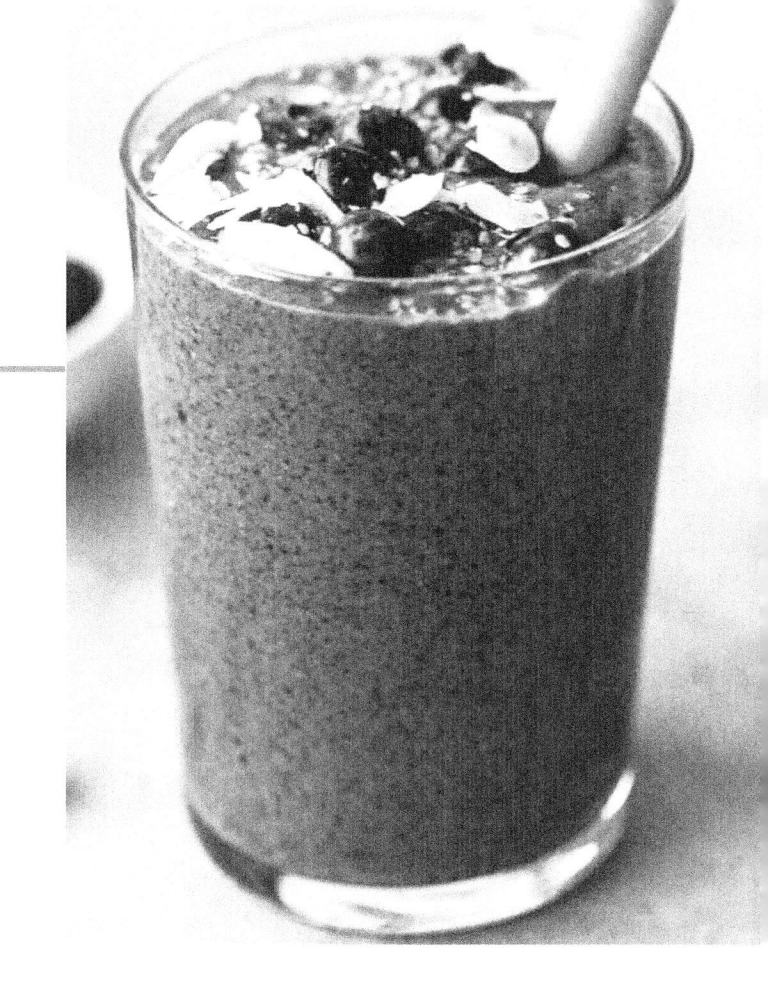

CHAPTER 09
SIDE DISHES

This section is built on a simple idea: the right side dish can turn an ordinary meal into something that supports your liver, satisfies your appetite, and helps your body work better—all without putting extra strain on digestion.

When managing liver cirrhosis, every part of the meal matters. Salads and side dishes offer a practical way to deliver nutrients without overwhelming the system. These recipes are light but filling. They focus on fiber, hydration, and natural flavor—without sodium, added fats, or processed ingredients. You'll find dishes built from fresh vegetables, legumes, grains, seeds, and heart-healthy oils. Nothing here is random. Each ingredient was selected to serve a specific purpose: reduce inflammation, support bile production, aid digestion, or provide slow-burning energy.

This isn't filler food. These are tools—flexible enough to stand alone for light meals or pair with the high-protein lunches and dinners from earlier sections. From warm bowls with roasted vegetables and lentils to crisp raw salads tossed with lemon juice and olive oil, everything here supports liver function and respects the challenges seniors face with chewing, swallowing, or energy dips.

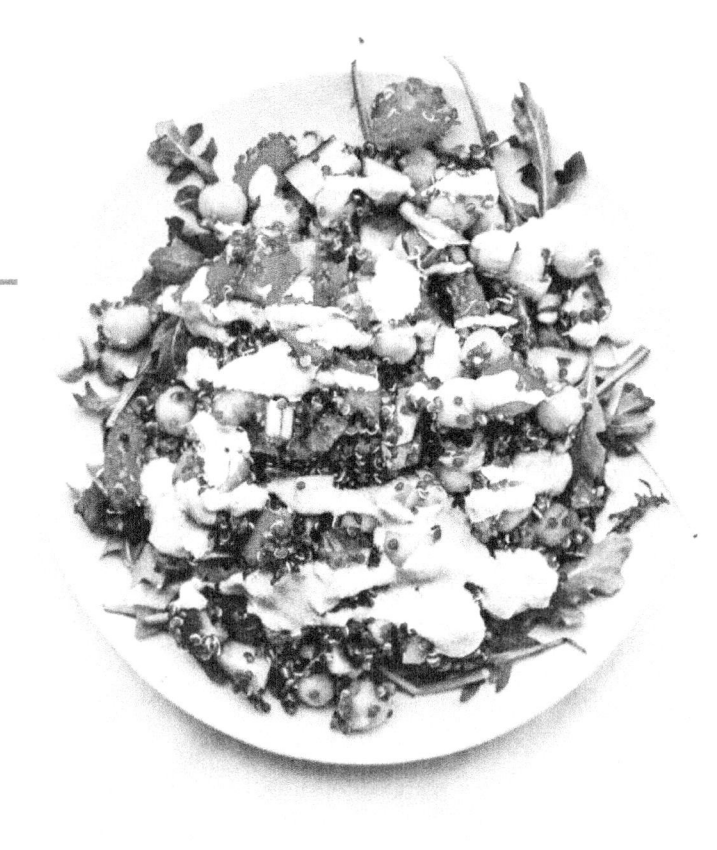

Quinoa Tabbouleh Salad

- **Preparation Time:** 20 minutes
- **Cooking Time:** 15 minutes
- **Servings:** 4

Ingredients:

- 1 cup quinoa
- 2 cups water
- 1 cup chopped parsley
- 1/2 cup chopped mint
- 2 tomatoes, diced
- 1 cucumber, diced
- 1/4 cup lemon juice
- 2 tablespoons olive oil
- Salt and pepper to taste

Instructions:

1. Rinse quinoa under cold water.
2. In a saucepan, combine quinoa and water. Bring to a boil, then simmer for 15 minutes until water is absorbed. Let it cool.
3. In a bowl, combine cooked quinoa, parsley, mint, tomatoes, and cucumber.
4. In a small bowl, whisk lemon juice, olive oil, salt, and pepper. Pour over quinoa mixture and toss well.

Portion per Day: 1 serving

Nutritional Values (per serving):

- **Calories:** 210 kcal
- **Protein:** 6 g
- **Carbohydrates:** 28 g
- **Fats:** 8 g
- **Fiber:** 5 g
- **Sodium:** 120 mg
- **Cholesterol:** 0 mg

Steamed Broccoli with Lemon-Garlic Dressing

- **Preparation Time:** 10 minutes
- **Cooking Time:** 10 minutes
- **Servings:** 4

Ingredients:

- 4 cups broccoli florets
- 2 tablespoons olive oil
- 2 cloves garlic, minced
- 1 tablespoon lemon juice
- Salt and pepper to taste

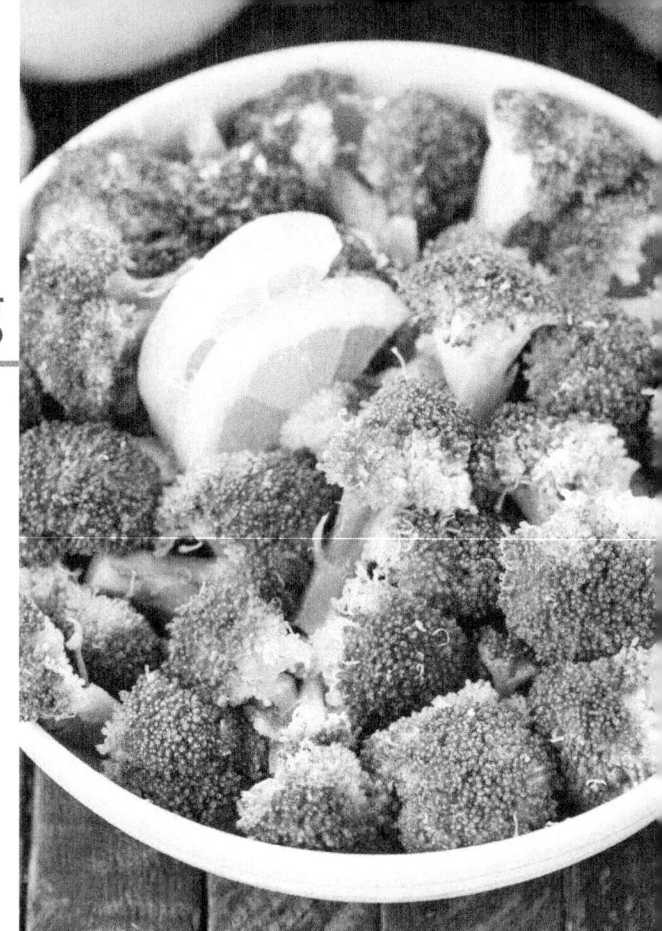

Instructions:

1. Steam broccoli florets for 5-7 minutes until tender-crisp.
2. In a small saucepan, heat olive oil over medium heat. Add minced garlic and sauté until fragrant.
3. Remove from heat and stir in lemon juice, salt, and pepper.
4. Drizzle dressing over steamed broccoli and serve.

Portion per Day: 1 serving

Nutritional Values (per serving):

- **Calories:** 120 kcal
- **Protein:** 4 g
- **Carbohydrates:** 10 g
- **Fats:** 8 g
- **Fiber:** 4 g
- **Sodium:** 80 mg
- **Cholesterol:** 0 mg

Citrus Avocado Salad

- **Preparation Time:** 10 minutes
- **Cooking Time:** 0 minutes
- **Servings:** 4

Ingredients:

- 1 avocado, sliced
- 1 orange, peeled and segmented
- 1/2 grapefruit, peeled and segmented
- 1 tablespoon olive oil
- 1 tablespoon fresh lemon juice
- Salt and pepper to taste

Instructions:

1. Arrange the avocado slices, orange segments, and grapefruit segments on a plate.
2. Drizzle with olive oil and fresh lemon juice.
3. Sprinkle with salt and pepper to taste.
4. Serve immediately as a refreshing, liver-friendly side dish.

Portion per Day: 1 serving

Nutritional Values (per serving):

- **Calories:** 160 kcal
- **Protein:** 2 g
- **Carbohydrates:** 15 g
- **Fats:** 12 g
- **Fiber:** 5 g
- **Sodium:** 60 mg
- **Cholesterol:** 0 mg

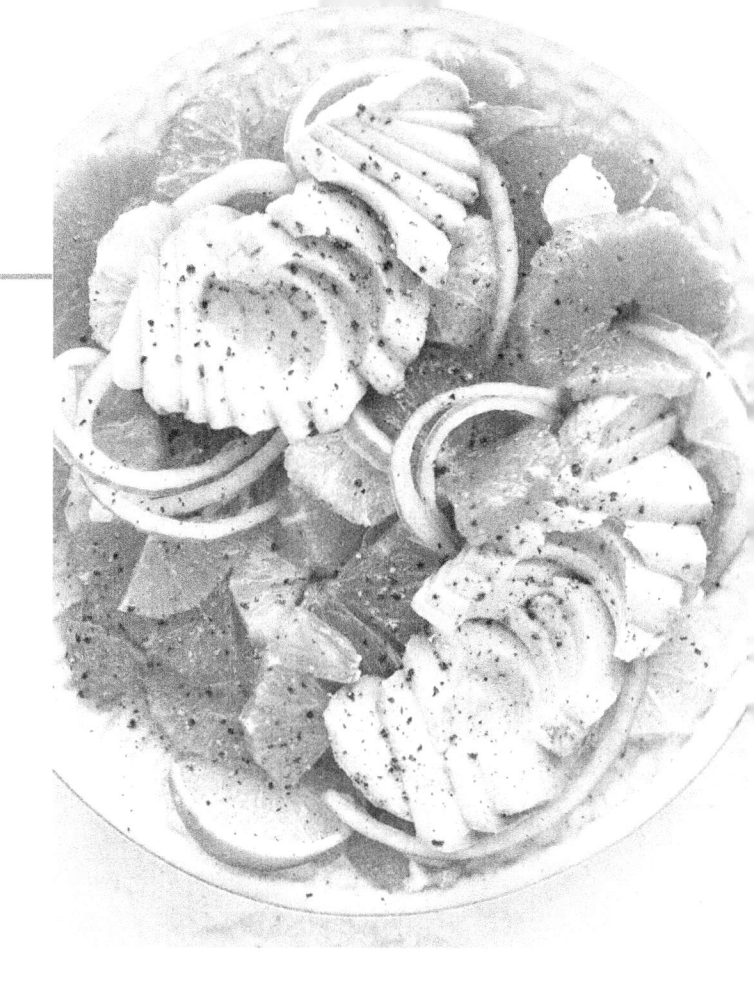

Garlic and Turmeric Roasted Vegetables

- **Preparation Time:** 10 minutes
- **Cooking Time:** 25 minutes
- **Servings:** 4

Ingredients:

- 1 cup cauliflower florets
- 1 cup broccoli florets
- 1 tablespoon olive oil
- 2 cloves garlic, minced
- 1/2 teaspoon turmeric powder
- Salt and pepper to taste

Instructions:

1. Preheat your oven to 400°F (200°C).
2. In a large bowl, toss the cauliflower and broccoli florets with olive oil, minced garlic, turmeric, salt, and pepper.
3. Spread the vegetables evenly on a baking sheet.
4. Roast for 20-25 minutes, or until the vegetables are tender and golden brown.
5. Serve warm as a flavorful side dish.

Portion per Day: 1 serving

Nutritional Values (per serving):

- **Calories:** 110 kcal
- **Protein:** 4 g
- **Carbohydrates:** 10 g
- **Fats:** 7 g
- **Fiber:** 4 g
- **Sodium:** 80 mg
- **Cholesterol:** 0 mg

Malfouf Salad (Lebanese Cabbage Salad)

- **Preparation Time:** 15 minutes
- **Cooking Time:** 0 minutes
- **Servings:** 4

Ingredients:

- 4 cups shredded cabbage
- 2 tablespoons lemon juice
- 2 tablespoons olive oil
- 2 cloves garlic, minced
- 1 teaspoon dried mint
- Salt to taste

Instructions:

1. In a large bowl, combine shredded cabbage and minced garlic.
2. In a small bowl, whisk together lemon juice, olive oil, dried mint, and salt.
3. Pour the dressing over the cabbage mixture and toss well.
4. Let it sit for 10 minutes to allow flavors to meld.
5. Serve as a refreshing side dish.

Portion per Day: 1 serving

Nutritional Values (per serving):

- **Calories:** 90 kcal
- **Protein:** 2 g
- **Carbohydrates:** 8 g
- **Fats:** 6 g
- **Fiber:** 3 g
- **Sodium:** 70 mg
- **Cholesterol:** 0 mg

Roasted Beet and Walnut Salad

- **Preparation Time:** 15 minutes
- **Cooking Time:** 40 minutes
- **Servings:** 4

Ingredients:

- 3 medium beets, peeled and diced
- 1 tablespoon olive oil
- 4 cups mixed greens
- 1/4 cup chopped walnuts
- 2 tablespoons balsamic vinegar
- Salt and pepper to taste

Instructions:

1. Preheat oven to 400°F (200°C).
2. Toss diced beets with olive oil, salt, and pepper. Spread on a baking sheet and roast for 35-40 minutes until tender.
3. In a large bowl, combine mixed greens, roasted beets, and walnuts.
4. Drizzle with balsamic vinegar and toss gently.
5. Serve as a nutritious side salad.

Portion per Day: 1 serving

Nutritional Values (per serving):

- **Calories:** 180 kcal
- **Protein:** 4 g
- **Carbohydrates:** 20 g
- **Fats:** 10 g
- **Fiber:** 5 g
- **Sodium:** 100 mg
- **Cholesterol:** 0 mg

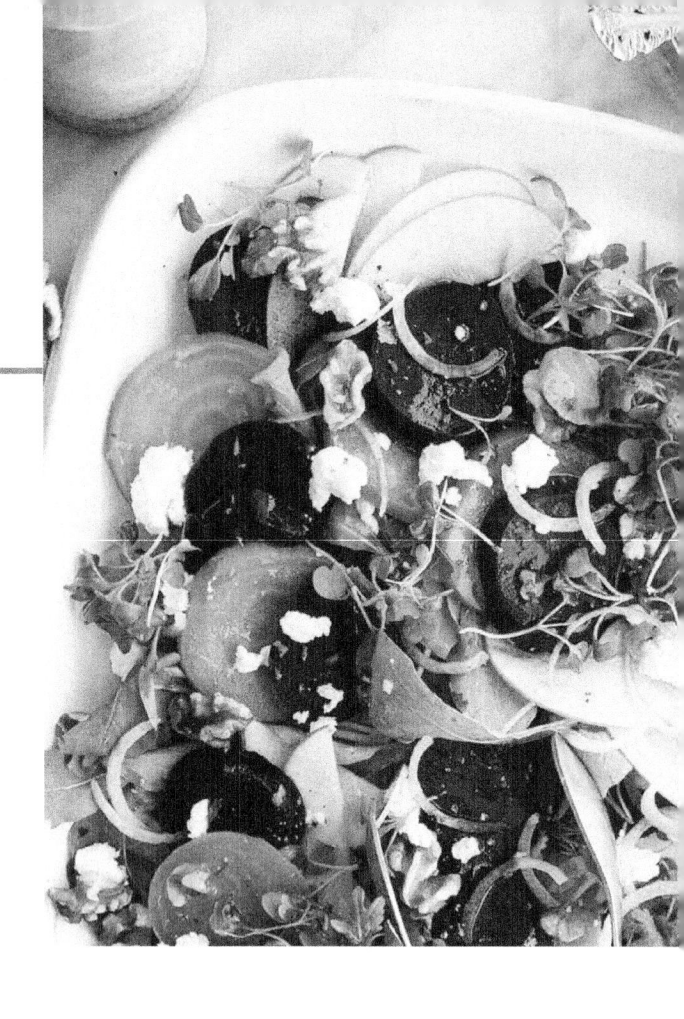

Warm Green Bean Salad

- **Preparation Time:** 10 minutes
- **Cooking Time:** 10 minutes
- **Servings:** 4

Ingredients:

- 4 cups green beans, trimmed
- 1 cup cherry tomatoes, halved
- 2 tablespoons olive oil
- 1 tablespoon lemon juice
- 2 cloves garlic, minced
- Salt and pepper to taste

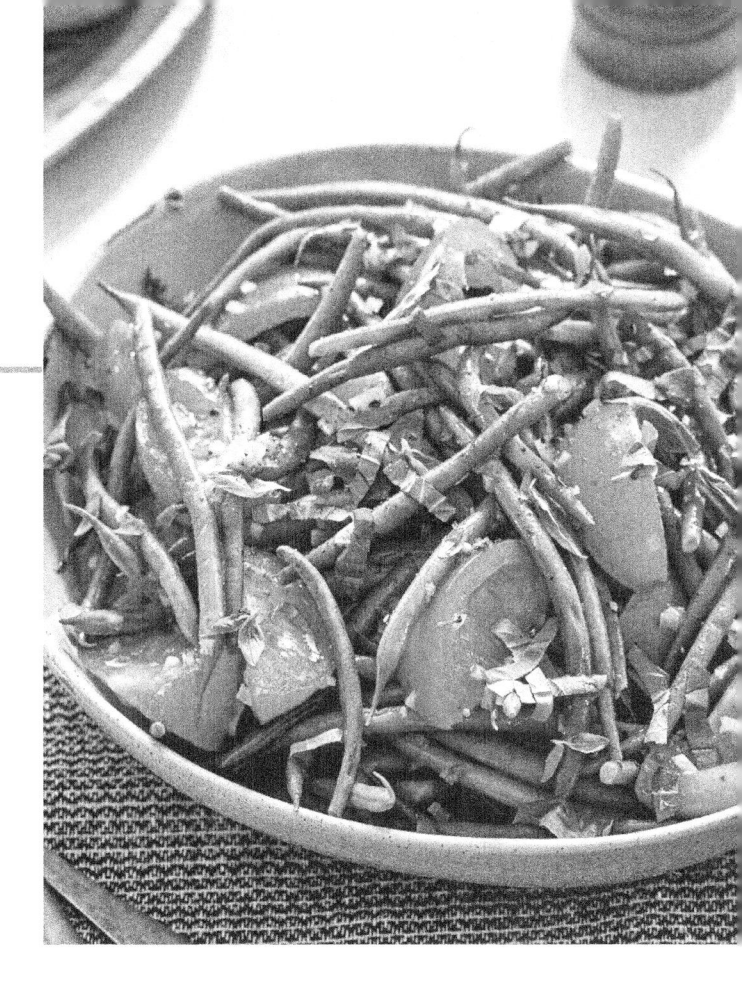

Instructions:

1. Steam green beans for 5-7 minutes until tender-crisp.
2. In a skillet, heat olive oil over medium heat. Add minced garlic and sauté until fragrant.
3. Add cherry tomatoes to the skillet and cook for 2-3 minutes.
4. Combine steamed green beans with the tomato mixture.
5. Drizzle with lemon juice, season with salt and pepper, and toss well.
6. Serve warm as a side dish.

Portion per Day: 1 serving

Nutritional Values (per serving):

- **Calories:** 120 kcal
- **Protein:** 3 g
- **Carbohydrates:** 12 g
- **Fats:** 7 g
- **Fiber:** 4 g
- **Sodium:** 90 mg
- **Cholesterol:** 0 mg

Grilled Asparagus with Lemon Zest

- **Preparation Time:** 10 minutes
- **Cooking Time:** 10 minutes
- **Servings:** 4

Ingredients:

- 1 bunch asparagus, trimmed
- 1 tablespoon olive oil
- 1 teaspoon lemon zest
- Salt and pepper to taste

Instructions:

1. Preheat grill to medium-high heat.
2. Toss asparagus with olive oil, salt, and pepper.
3. Grill asparagus for 5-7 minutes, turning occasionally, until tender and slightly charred.
4. Remove from grill and sprinkle with lemon zest before serving.

Portion per Day: 1 serving

Nutritional Values (per serving):

- **Calories:** 80 kcal
- **Protein:** 3 g
- **Carbohydrates:** 5 g
- **Fats:** 6 g
- **Fiber:** 3 g
- **Sodium:** 50 mg
- **Cholesterol:** 0 mg

Carrot and Raisin Salad

- **Preparation Time:** 15 minutes
- **Cooking Time:** 0 minutes
- **Servings:** 4

Ingredients:

- 2 cups shredded carrots
- 1/2 cup raisins
- 1/4 cup plain Greek yogurt
- 1 tablespoon honey
- 1 tablespoon lemon juice
- 1/4 teaspoon cinnamon

Instructions:

1. In a large bowl, combine shredded carrots and raisins.
2. In a small bowl, mix Greek yogurt, honey, lemon juice, and cinnamon until well combined.
3. Pour the dressing over the carrot mixture and toss to coat evenly.
4. Chill for 30 minutes before serving.

Portion per Day: 1 serving

Nutritional Values (per serving):

- **Calories:** 150 kcal
- **Protein:** 3 g
- **Carbohydrates:** 25 g
- **Fats:** 4 g
- **Fiber:** 3 g
- **Sodium:** 45 mg
- **Cholesterol:** 2 mg

Spinach and Strawberry Salad

- **Preparation Time:** 10 minutes
- **Cooking Time:** 0 minutes
- **Servings:** 4

Ingredients:

- 4 cups baby spinach
- 1 cup sliced strawberries
- 1/4 cup sliced almonds
- 2 tablespoons balsamic vinegar
- 1 tablespoon olive oil
- Salt and pepper to taste

Instructions:

1. In a large bowl, combine baby spinach, sliced strawberries, and sliced almonds.
2. In a small bowl, whisk together balsamic vinegar, olive oil, salt, and pepper.
3. Drizzle the dressing over the salad and toss gently to combine.
4. Serve immediately.

Portion per Day: 1 serving

Nutritional Values (per serving):

- **Calories:** 140 kcal
- **Protein:** 3 g
- **Carbohydrates:** 10 g
- **Fats:** 10 g
- **Fiber:** 3 g
- **Sodium:** 50 mg
- **Cholesterol:** 0 mg

Artichoke and Cashew Detox Salad

- **Preparation Time:** 15 minutes
- **Cooking Time:** 0 minutes
- **Servings:** 4

Ingredients:

- 1 can (15 oz) artichoke hearts, drained and chopped
- 1/2 cup raw cashews
- 2 cups arugula
- 1/4 cup chopped fresh parsley
- 1/4 cup thinly sliced red onion
- 2 tablespoons lemon juice
- 1 tablespoon red wine vinegar
- 1 tablespoon olive oil
- Salt and pepper to taste

Instructions:

1. In a large bowl, combine artichoke hearts, cashews, arugula, parsley, and red onion.
2. In a small bowl, whisk together lemon juice, red wine vinegar, olive oil, salt, and pepper.
3. Pour dressing over the salad and toss to combine.
4. Refrigerate for 20 minutes before serving to allow flavors to meld.

Portion per Day: 1 serving

Nutritional Values (per serving):

- **Calories:** 220 kcal
- **Protein:** 5 g
- **Carbohydrates:** 12 g
- **Fats:** 16 g
- **Fiber:** 4 g
- **Sodium:** 140 mg
- **Cholesterol:** 0 mg

CHAPTER 10 BONUS

Lifestyle Tips for Managing Liver Cirrhosis

Gentle Exercise Recommendations for Seniors

Staying active helps your liver and your whole body. It improves circulation, boosts mood, supports digestion, and preserves muscle—something many seniors with cirrhosis struggle to maintain. Regular movement also helps manage fatigue and supports balance, which lowers the risk of falls.

Cirrhosis often brings tiredness, swelling, and discomfort. That doesn't mean you should stop moving. It means your approach to exercise needs to change. You don't need a gym. You don't need equipment. You need routines that are gentle, safe, and regular.

Benefits of Exercise for Seniors with Cirrhosis

- Maintains muscle mass and strength
- Improves balance and mobility
- Aids digestion and reduces bloating
- Lowers anxiety and depression
- Supports healthy weight and blood sugar
- Improves sleep quality

Recommended Exercises

1. Walking

- Easiest and most accessible
- Start with 5–10 minutes a day
- Add 1–2 minutes each week as tolerated
- Use a cane or walker for stability
- Walk indoors if weather is poor

2. Seated or Chair Exercises

- Great for those with limited energy or mobility
- Include:
    - Arm circles
    - Seated marches
    - Knee lifts
    - Light resistance band pulls
- Perform in short sets (1–2 minutes at a time)

3. Gentle Stretching

- Increases flexibility and range of motion
- Focus on neck, shoulders, back, and legs
- Breathe slowly and move without forcing
- Helps reduce stiffness and morning aches

4. Tai Chi and Gentle Yoga

- Slow, flowing movements
- Boosts balance, focus, and coordination
- Can be adapted with chair support
- Avoid deep twists or poses that strain the abdomen

5. Water-Based Exercise

- Swimming or water aerobics reduce joint stress
- The water supports your body and reduces swelling
- Always go with someone if fatigue or cramps are a concern

Tips for Safe Activity

- Talk to your doctor first, especially if you have ascites or low energy
- Start slow and rest when needed
- Avoid high-impact moves
- Stay hydrated before and after
- Wear supportive shoes
- Schedule activity during your most energetic time of day
- Stop if you feel dizzy, short of breath, or confused

Mental Well-Being and Stress Management

Seniors with cirrhosis often face stress, sadness, and frustration. These feelings are real. They matter. Left unchecked, they affect appetite, sleep, and healing. Mental well-being is just as important as stress

Common Challenges

- Fear about your future
- Frustration over diet changes
- Isolation from friends and family
- Fatigue that limits social life
- Sleep problems or memory changes

Strategies That Help

1. Structure Your Day

- Create a simple routine
- Eat meals at the same time
- Set small, daily goals
- Include time for rest and activity

2. Stay Connected

- Call or visit a friend each week
- Join a support group (in-person or online)
- Share meals with family
- Let others help with shopping or cooking

3. Focus on What You Control

- Choose foods that help your liver
- Stick to movement you can handle
- Track how you feel each day
- Celebrate consistency, not perfection

4. Practice Simple Relaxation

- Try deep breathing (inhale 4, hold 4, exhale 4)
- Listen to calming music
- Sit in a quiet room for 10 minutes
- Try light stretching or a short walk

5. Talk to Someone

- Speak to a counselor, doctor, or support group
- Tell someone if you feel hopeless
- Don't wait for a crisis—reach out early

6. Get Outside

- Sit in the sun for 10–15 minutes
- Walk around the block
- Breathe fresh air

90-Day Meal Plan

Day	Breakfast	Lunch	Dinner
1	Egg White and Veggie Scramble with Toast (p.35)	Grilled Shrimp and Quinoa Bowl (p.40)	Lemon Herb Grilled Chicken with Steamed Broccoli (p.60)
2	Vegetable Breakfast Wrap (p.23)	Baked Salmon with Dill Yogurt Sauce (p.44)	Stuffed Zucchini Boats (p.67)
3	Sweet Potato and Egg Hash (p.19)	Grilled Shrimp and Quinoa Bowl (p.40)	Chard and Mushroom Frittata (p.77)
4	Greek Yogurt Parfait with Berries and Nuts (p.17)	Red Lentil and Carrot Soup (p.55)	Zucchini Noodles with Pesto and Cherry Tomatoes (p.73)
5	Oatmeal with Berries and Flaxseed (p.16)	Quinoa and Black Bean Bowl (p.37)	Quinoa and Black Bean Stuffed Peppers (p.62)
6	Banana Oat Pancakes (p.21)	Baked Salmon with Dill Yogurt Sauce (p.44)	Vegetable Buckwheat Bowl with Tahini Sauce (p.76)
7	Cottage Cheese & Berry Wrap (p.34)	Quinoa and Black Bean Bowl (p.37)	Chard and Mushroom Frittata (p.77)
8	Banana Oat Pancakes (p.21)	Tempeh and Veggie Stir Fry (p.57)	Chard and Mushroom Frittata (p.77)
9	Sweet Potato and Black Bean Hash (p.28)	Baked Salmon with Dill Yogurt Sauce (p.44)	Cauliflower and Chickpea Curry (p.74)
10	Smoothie with Spinach, Banana, and Flaxseed (p.33)	Chickpea and Spinach Stew (p.45)	Lemon Herb Grilled Chicken with Steamed Broccoli (p.60)
11	Spinach and Mushroom Omelette (p.20)	Chickpea and Avocado Lettuce Wraps (p.50)	Grilled Turkey Burger with Avocado Spread (p.70)
12	Vegetable Breakfast Wrap (p.23)	Lentil and Sweet Potato Stew (p.41)	Grilled Chicken Salad with Avocado (p.66)
13	Avocado and Tomato Toast (p.25)	Grilled Shrimp and Quinoa Bowl (p.40)	Quinoa and Black Bean Stuffed Peppers (p.62)
14	Tofu Scramble (p.27)	Grilled Shrimp and Quinoa Bowl (p.40)	Baked Eggplant Parmesan (p.71)
15	Berry Smoothie Bowl (p.26)	Edamame and Barley Power Bowl (p.56)	Quinoa and Chickpea Salad (p.68)
16	Oatmeal with Berries and Flaxseed (p.16)	Turkey and Spinach Stuffed Bell Peppers (p.51)	Chard and Mushroom Frittata (p.77)
17	Quinoa Breakfast Bowl (p.18)	Baked Cod with Lemon and Dill (p.49)	Quinoa and Black Bean Stuffed Peppers (p.62)

Day	Breakfast	Lunch	Dinner
18	Oatmeal with Sliced Apples and Cinnamon (p.32)	Lentil and Vegetable Soup (p.46)	Baked Eggplant Parmesan (p.71)
19	Smoothie with Spinach, Banana, and Flaxseed (p.33)	Eggplant and Chickpea Stir-Fry (p.43)	Quinoa and Black Bean Stuffed Peppers (p.62)
20	Oatmeal with Berries and Flaxseed (p.16)	Baked Falafel with Cucumber Yogurt Dip (p.58)	Stuffed Zucchini Boats (p.67)
21	Apple Cinnamon Quinoa (p.24)	Lentil and Quinoa Salad (p.39)	Stuffed Zucchini Boats (p.67)
22	Quinoa Breakfast Bowl (p.18)	Baked Cod with Lemon and Dill (p.49)	Quinoa and Chickpea Salad (p.68)
23	Greek Yogurt with Walnuts and Honey (p.29)	Tempeh and Veggie Stir Fry (p.57)	Baked Eggplant Parmesan (p.71)
24	Spinach and Mushroom Omelette (p.20)	Grilled Chicken and Quinoa Salad (p.48)	Baked Eggplant Parmesan (p.71)
25	Banana Oat Pancakes (p.21)	Baked Falafel with Cucumber Yogurt Dip (p.58)	Quinoa and Chickpea Salad (p.68)
26	Egg White and Veggie Scramble with Toast (p.35)	Lentil and Quinoa Salad (p.39)	Quinoa and Vegetable Stir-Fry (p.65)
27	Oatmeal with Sliced Apples and Cinnamon (p.32)	Baked Salmon with Dill Yogurt Sauce (p.44)	Quinoa and Vegetable Stir-Fry (p.65)
28	Greek Yogurt with Walnuts and Honey (p.29)	Baked Cod with Lemon and Dill (p.49)	Quinoa and Chickpea Salad (p.68)
29	Egg White and Veggie Scramble with Toast (p.35)	Grilled Chicken and Cucumber Wrap (p.54)	Stuffed Zucchini Boats (p.67)
30	Avocado and Tomato Toast (p.25)	Turkey and Avocado Wrap (p.38)	Stuffed Zucchini Boats (p.67)
31	Oatmeal with Berries and Flaxseed (p.16)	Grilled Tofu and Vegetable Skewers (p.47)	Shrimp and Vegetable Stir-Fry (p.72)
32	Vegetable Breakfast Wrap (p.23)	Lentil and Quinoa Salad (p.39)	Grilled Chicken Salad with Avocado (p.66)

Day	Breakfast	Lunch	Dinner
33	Smoothie with Spinach, Banana, and Flaxseed (p.33)	Grilled Tofu and Vegetable Skewers (p.47)	Grilled Chicken Salad with Avocado (p.66)
34	Egg White and Veggie Scramble with Toast (p.35)	Tofu Stir-Fry with Brown Rice (p.52)	Shrimp and Vegetable Stir-Fry (p.72)
35	Egg White and Veggie Scramble with Toast (p.35)	Turkey and Spinach Stuffed Bell Peppers (p.51)	Baked Tilapia with Lemon and Herbs (p.64)
36	Vegetable Breakfast Wrap (p.23)	Lentil and Sweet Potato Stew (p.41)	Stuffed Zucchini Boats (p.67)
37	Oatmeal with Sliced Apples and Cinnamon (p.32)	Grilled Chicken and Cucumber Wrap (p.54)	Quinoa and Chickpea Salad (p.68)
38	Smoothie with Spinach, Banana, and Flaxseed (p.33)	Chickpea and Avocado Lettuce Wraps (p.50)	Grilled Seitan and Cabbage Slaw Wrap (p.78)
39	Tofu Scramble (p.27)	Grilled Chicken and Quinoa Salad (p.48)	Stuffed Zucchini Boats (p.67)
40	Sweet Potato and Egg Hash (p.19)	Sardine and Avocado Whole Grain Sandwich (p.53)	Seared Scallops with Spinach and Millet (p.75)
41	Greek Yogurt Parfait with Berries and Nuts (p.17)	Turkey and Avocado Wrap (p.38)	Grilled Salmon with Spinach and Brown Rice (p.63)
42	Sweet Potato and Egg Hash (p.19)	Tempeh and Veggie Stir Fry (p.57)	Quinoa and Vegetable Stir-Fry (p.65)
43	Sweet Potato and Black Bean Hash (p.28)	Edamame and Barley Power Bowl (p.56)	Quinoa and Black Bean Stuffed Peppers (p.62)
44	Tofu Scramble (p.27)	Baked Cod with Lemon and Dill (p.49)	Cauliflower and Chickpea Curry (p.74)
45	Vegetable and Tofu Stir-Fry (p.31)	Chickpea and Spinach Stew (p.45)	Chard and Mushroom Frittata (p.77)
46	Berry Chia Pudding (p.15)	Baked Falafel with Cucumber Yogurt Dip (p.58)	Grilled Salmon with Spinach and Brown Rice (p.63)
47	Oatmeal with Sliced Apples and Cinnamon (p.32)	Chickpea and Spinach Stew (p.45)	Grilled Turkey Burger with Avocado Spread (p.70)
48	Quinoa Breakfast Bowl (p.18)	Lentil and Vegetable Soup (p.46)	Zucchini Noodles with Pesto and Cherry Tomatoes (p.73)

Day	Breakfast	Lunch	Dinner
49	Spinach and Mushroom Omelette (p.20)	Turkey and Spinach Stuffed Bell Peppers (p.51)	Lemon Herb Grilled Chicken with Steamed Broccoli (p.60)
50	Vegetable Breakfast Wrap (p.23)	Sardine and Avocado Whole Grain Sandwich (p.53)	Quinoa and Vegetable Stir-Fry (p.65)
51	Vegetable and Tofu Stir-Fry (p.31)	Grilled Shrimp and Quinoa Bowl (p.40)	Grilled Portobello Mushrooms with Brown Rice (p.69)
52	Egg White and Veggie Scramble with Toast (p.35)	Sardine and Avocado Whole Grain Sandwich (p.53)	Grilled Chicken Salad with Avocado (p.66)
53	Sweet Potato and Egg Hash (p.19)	Grilled Chicken and Quinoa Salad (p.48)	Quinoa and Vegetable Stir-Fry (p.65)
54	Oatmeal with Sliced Apples and Cinnamon (p.32)	Sardine and Avocado Whole Grain Sandwich (p.53)	Lemon Herb Grilled Chicken with Steamed Broccoli (p.60)
55	Cottage Cheese & Berry Wrap (p.34)	Grilled Tofu and Vegetable Skewers (p.47)	Seared Scallops with Spinach and Millet (p.75)
56	Berry Chia Pudding (p.15)	Grilled Shrimp and Quinoa Bowl (p.40)	Baked Eggplant Parmesan (p.71)
57	Apple Cinnamon Quinoa (p.24)	Baked Salmon with Dill Yogurt Sauce (p.44)	Baked Cod with Quinoa and Asparagus (p.61)
58	Cottage Cheese with Pineapple (p.22)	Red Lentil and Carrot Soup (p.55)	Quinoa and Black Bean Stuffed Peppers (p.62)
59	Greek Yogurt Parfait with Berries and Nuts (p.17)	Tofu Stir-Fry with Brown Rice (p.52)	Quinoa and Black Bean Stuffed Peppers (p.62)
60	Oatmeal with Sliced Apples and Cinnamon (p.32)	Lentil and Sweet Potato Stew (p.41)	Baked Tilapia with Lemon and Herbs (p.64)
61	Whole Grain Toast with Almond Butter and Banana (p.30)	Grilled Chicken and Cucumber Wrap (p.54)	Quinoa and Vegetable Stir-Fry (p.65)
62	Vegetable Breakfast Wrap (p.23)	Sardine and Avocado Whole Grain Sandwich (p.53)	Zucchini Noodles with Pesto and Cherry Tomatoes (p.73)
63	Banana Oat Pancakes (p.21)	Grilled Chicken and Cucumber Wrap (p.54)	Grilled Chicken Salad with Avocado (p.66)

Day	Breakfast	Lunch	Dinner
64	Apple Cinnamon Quinoa (p.24)	Baked Cod with Lemon and Dill (p.49)	Baked Eggplant Parmesan (p.71)
65	Greek Yogurt with Walnuts and Honey (p.29)	Sardine and Avocado Whole Grain Sandwich (p.53)	Cauliflower and Chickpea Curry (p.74)
66	Quinoa Breakfast Bowl (p.18)	Baked Salmon with Dill Yogurt Sauce (p.44)	Stuffed Zucchini Boats (p.67)
67	Greek Yogurt Parfait with Berries and Nuts (p.17)	Grilled Tofu and Vegetable Skewers (p.47)	Lemon Herb Grilled Chicken with Steamed Broccoli (p.60)
68	Smoothie with Spinach, Banana, and Flaxseed (p.33)	Grilled Chicken and Cucumber Wrap (p.54)	Stuffed Zucchini Boats (p.67)
69	Smoothie with Spinach, Banana, and Flaxseed (p.33)	Baked Salmon with Dill Yogurt Sauce (p.44)	Lemon Herb Grilled Chicken with Steamed Broccoli (p.60)
70	Greek Yogurt Parfait with Berries and Nuts (p.17)	Tempeh and Veggie Stir Fry (p.57)	Baked Cod with Quinoa and Asparagus (p.61)
71	Cottage Cheese with Pineapple (p.22)	Lentil and Quinoa Salad (p.39)	Baked Cod with Quinoa and Asparagus (p.61)
72	Avocado and Tomato Toast (p.25)	Lentil and Quinoa Salad (p.39)	Vegetable Buckwheat Bowl with Tahini Sauce (p.76)
73	Cottage Cheese with Pineapple (p.22)	Chickpea and Spinach Stew (p.45)	Seared Scallops with Spinach and Millet (p.75)
74	Banana Oat Pancakes (p.21)	Grilled Chicken and Cucumber Wrap (p.54)	Baked Tilapia with Lemon and Herbs (p.64)
75	Smoothie with Spinach, Banana, and Flaxseed (p.33)	Red Lentil and Carrot Soup (p.55)	Seared Scallops with Spinach and Millet (p.75)
76	Cottage Cheese with Pineapple (p.22)	Tofu Stir-Fry with Brown Rice (p.52)	Zucchini Noodles with Pesto and Cherry Tomatoes (p.73)
77	Banana Oat Pancakes (p.21)	Grilled Shrimp and Quinoa Bowl (p.40)	Grilled Salmon with Spinach and Brown Rice (p.63)
78	Sweet Potato and Black Bean Hash (p.28)	Grilled Chicken and Quinoa Salad (p.48)	Zucchini Noodles with Pesto and Cherry Tomatoes (p.73)

Day	Breakfast	Lunch	Dinner
79	Sweet Potato and Black Bean Hash (p.28)	Turkey and Spinach Stuffed Bell Peppers (p.51)	Baked Cod with Quinoa and Asparagus (p.61)
80	Egg White and Veggie Scramble with Toast (p.35)	Tempeh and Veggie Stir Fry (p.57)	Grilled Salmon with Spinach and Brown Rice (p.63)
81	Oatmeal with Berries and Flaxseed (p.16)	Baked Cod with Lemon and Dill (p.49)	Grilled Turkey Burger with Avocado Spread (p.70)
82	Quinoa Breakfast Bowl (p.18)	Baked Salmon with Dill Yogurt Sauce (p.44)	Grilled Chicken Salad with Avocado (p.66)
83	Banana Oat Pancakes (p.21)	Grilled Chicken and Cucumber Wrap (p.54)	Cauliflower and Chickpea Curry (p.74)
84	Sweet Potato and Egg Hash (p.19)	Chickpea and Avocado Lettuce Wraps (p.50)	Quinoa and Vegetable Stir-Fry (p.65)
85	Vegetable Breakfast Wrap (p.23)	Turkey and Spinach Stuffed Bell Peppers (p.51)	Stuffed Zucchini Boats (p.67)
86	Greek Yogurt Parfait with Berries and Nuts (p.17)	Turkey and Spinach Stuffed Bell Peppers (p.51)	Chard and Mushroom Frittata (p.77)
87	Quinoa Breakfast Bowl (p.18)	Turkey and Avocado Wrap (p.38)	Chard and Mushroom Frittata (p.77)
88	Berry Chia Pudding (p.15)	Lentil and Quinoa Salad (p.39)	Stuffed Zucchini Boats (p.67)
89	Spinach and Mushroom Omelette (p.20)	Chickpea and Avocado Lettuce Wraps (p.50)	Seared Scallops with Spinach and Millet (p.75)
90	Whole Grain Toast with Almond Butter and Banana (p.30)	Eggplant and Chickpea Stir-Fry (p.43)	Shrimp and Vegetable Stir-Fry (p.72)

Monthly Shopping List

Month 1

Vegetables

spinach	6 cups
tomato	4 units
onion	4 units
bell pepper	3 units
zucchini	3 units
chard	2 cups
mushrooms	2 cups
broccoli	2 heads
carrot	3 units
garlic	4 cloves
cherry tomatoes	1 cup

Fruits

avocado	2 units
berries	3 cups
lemon	2 units
lime	1 unit

Dairy & Alternatives

greek yogurt	2 cups
almond milk	2 cups

Wraps & Bread

whole grain bread	6 slices
whole grain tortilla	2 units

Grains & Legumes

quinoa	3 cups
black beans	2 cups
corn	1 cup
red lentils	2 cups
oats	2 cups

Proteins

egg	8 units
egg whites	6 units
shrimp	1 lb
salmon	2 fillets
chicken breast	2 lbs
cheese	1 cup

Herbs & Condiments

olive oil	1 cup
dill	1 tbsp
honey	2 tbsp
herbs	1 bunch
basil	1 bunch

Nuts & Seeds

flaxseed	2 tbsp
nuts	1/2 cup

Month 2

Vegetables

spinach	8 cups
tomato	2 units
onion	4 units
bell pepper	4 units
zucchini	3 units
carrot	3 units
broccoli	2 heads
garlic	2 cloves

Fruits

banana	2 units
berries	2 cups
avocado	2 units
lemon	2 units

Grains & Legumes

quinoa	2 cups
lentils	2 cups
brown rice	2 cups
oats	2 cups

Proteins

egg	4 units
egg whites	6 units
tofu	3 blocks
shrimp	1 lb
chicken breast	2 lbs
ground turkey	1 lb
tilapia	2 fillets

Dairy & Alternatives

almond milk	2 cups

Herbs & Condiments

olive oil	1 cup
herbs	1 bunch

Nuts & Seeds

flaxseed	2 tbsp

Wraps & Bread

whole grain bread	4 slices
whole grain tortilla	2 units

Month 3

Vegetables

spinach	14 cup
onion	9 unit
bell pepper	4 unit
zucchini	6 unit
mushrooms	2 cup
garlic	5 clove
tomato	3 unit
cucumber	1 unit
eggplant	2 unit
asparagus	1 bunch
cauliflower	1 head

Fruits

banana	4 unit
apple	1 unit
avocado	6 unit
lemon	9 unit

Wraps & Bread

whole grain bread	8 slice
whole grain tortilla	3 unit

Dairy & Alternatives

greek yogurt	1.5 cup
cottage cheese	0.5 cup
almond milk	6 cup

Grains & Legumes

Quinoa	4.5 cup
oats	1.0 cup
brown rice	2 unit
red lentils	0.5 cup
black beans	0.5 cup

Proteins

egg	5 unit
egg whites	1 unit
chicken breast	2.0 lb
shrimp	8 oz
salmon	2 fillet
cod	2 fillet
scallops	3 oz
sardines	1 can
ground turkey	1.0 lb

Condiments & Oils

olive oil	27 tbsp
honey	2 tbsp
dill	1.0 tbsp
basil	1 bunch

Nuts & Seeds

almond butter	1 tbsp
flaxseed	2 tbsp
nuts	0.25 cup

CONCLUSION

Managing liver cirrhosis through diet is not about restrictions—it's about making choices that support your body every day. This cookbook has shown that healthy meals can be simple, satisfying, and suited to the needs of seniors. You've seen how breakfast, lunch, dinner, and even snacks can be high in protein, low in sodium, and gentle on the liver.

By following these recipes, you're not only feeding yourself—you're actively caring for your liver. Choosing whole foods over processed ones, limiting salt and fat, and staying hydrated aren't trends. They're habits that protect your health long-term.

This isn't a temporary fix. It's a way of eating that helps reduce symptoms, supports your energy, and fits your routine. The tools are here—meal plans, shopping lists, easy instructions—so you don't have to guess.

The lifestyle changes may feel small, but the impact is steady. One meal at a time, you're building something stronger. Stay consistent. Be patient with yourself. Your liver will thank you

Ingredient Substitution Chart

Here is a practical Ingredient Substitution Chart tailored for a liver-healthy diet. It replaces common problematic ingredients with options that are easier on the liver, lower in sodium, and support better digestion and nutrient absorption.

Ingredient to Avoid	Liver-Healthy Substitute	Why It's Better
Table Salt	Lemon juice, herbs, garlic, onion	Enhances flavor without increasing blood pressure
Butter	Olive oil, avocado, mashed banana	Lower in saturated fat; supports heart and liver health
Red meat (beef, lamb)	Skinless chicken, turkey, tofu, lentils	Reduces fat intake; easier to digest
Whole milk	Unsweetened almond or oat milk	Lower in fat; lactose-free
Heavy cream	Greek yogurt, blended silken tofu	High in protein; low in saturated fat
Processed meats (bacon, ham)	Grilled chicken breast, homemade falafel	Avoids preservatives and sodium
White rice	Brown rice, quinoa, barley	Higher in fiber and nutrients
White bread	Whole grain bread, sprouted grain bread	Stabilizes blood sugar; more nutrients
Fried foods	Baked, grilled, or steamed alternatives	Reduces fat and inflammatory load
Store-bought dressings	Olive oil + lemon/vinegar + herbs	No added sugars or sodium
Sugar (refined)	Stevia, mashed fruit, date paste	Avoids blood sugar spikes
Canned soups	Homemade vegetable or lentil soup	Lower sodium, cleaner ingredients
Alcohol (wine, beer, spirits)	Infused water, herbal tea	Completely avoids liver-damaging effects
Full-fat cheese	Low-fat cottage cheese or ricotta	Less saturated fat, easier on liver
Mayonnaise	Mashed avocado, hummus, plain yogurt	Heart-healthy fats; nutrient-dense

FREE CONSULTATION

Dear Reader,

Thank you for purchasing my cookbook! To enhance your culinary journey, I'm offering a complimentary email consultation to personalize these recipes for your specific needs and kitchen setup.

Whether you need advice on ingredient substitutions, guidance adapting recipes for dietary restrictions, or recommendations for techniques compatible with your equipment, I'm delighted to assist.

To access this service, email me at seraphinamercer.diets11@gmail.com with "**Cookbook Consultation**" in the subject line, briefly describing your question. You'll receive personalized cooking advice within **48 hours**.

This exclusive benefit is reserved for cookbook purchasers only.

Happy cooking—I look forward to helping you bring these recipes to life in your kitchen!

Thank you for choosing

" The Complete Liver Cirrhosis Diet Cookbook for Seniors 2025

by

Seraphina Mercer"

To enhance your experience, we've designed a "**Printable Weekly Meal Plan**" that organizes and simplifies your weekly food preparation, supporting your wellness journey every step of the way.

Embrace your path toward better health, renewed strength, and deeper relaxation.

Index

A

Apple Cinnamon Quinoa, 24

Apple Pie Oatmeal Cookies, 81

Apple-Celery Liver Cleanser, 103

Artichoke and Cashew Detox Salad, 119

Avocado & Spinach Smoothie, 98

Avocado and Tomato Toast, 25

Avocado Chocolate Mousse, 83

Avocado-Cilantro Smoothie, 100

B

Baked Apple Chips, 86

Baked Cinnamon Pears, 84

Baked Cod with Lemon and Dill, 49

Baked Cod with Quinoa and Asparagus, 61

Baked Eggplant Parmesan, 71

Baked Falafel with Cucumber Yogurt Dip, 58

Baked Salmon with Dill Yogurt Sauce, 44

Baked Sweet Potato Chips, 91

Baked Tilapia with Lemon and Herbs, 64

Baked Zucchini Fries, 88

Banana Oat Pancakes, 21

Beetroot & Berry Detox Smoothie, 94

Beetroot & Carrot Juice, 105

Berry Chia Pudding, 15

Berry Smoothie Bowl, 26

Berry-Lemon Infused Water, 101

Black Bean Brownies, 80

Blueberry & Avocado Smoothie, 107

C

Carrot and Oat Energy Bites, 85

Carrot and Raisin Salad, 117

Carrot-Apple Detox Juice, 99

Cauliflower and Chickpea Curry, 74

Chard and Mushroom Frittata, 77

Chia and Raspberry Jam, 89

Chickpea and Avocado Lettuce Wraps, 50

Chickpea and Spinach Stew, 45

Citrus Avocado Salad, 111

Coconut Water & Chia Refresher, 102

Cottage Cheese & Berry Wrap, 34

Cottage Cheese with Pineapple, 22

Cucumber & Mint Cooler, 97

E & F

Edamame and Barley Power Bowl, 56

Egg White and Veggie Scramble with Toast, 35

Eggplant and Chickpea Stir-Fry, 43

Frozen Banana Bites, 92

G

Garlic and Turmeric Roasted Vegetables, 112

Grapefruit & Kefir Smoothie, 104

Greek Yogurt Parfait with Berries and Nuts, 17

Greek Yogurt with Walnuts and Honey, 29

Green Tea & Citrus Refresher, 95

Grilled Asparagus with Lemon Zest, 116

Grilled Chicken and Cucumber Wrap, 54

Grilled Chicken and Quinoa Salad, 48

Grilled Chicken Salad with Avocado, 66

Grilled Portobello Mushrooms with Brown Rice, 69

Grilled Salmon with Spinach and Brown Rice, 63

Grilled Seitan and Cabbage Slaw Wrap, 78

Grilled Shrimp and Quinoa Bowl, 40

Grilled Tofu and Vegetable Skewers, 47

Grilled Turkey and Zucchini Skewers, 42

Grilled Turkey Burger with Avocado Spread, 70

L

Lemon Herb Grilled Chicken with Steamed Broccoli, 60

Lentil and Quinoa Salad, 39

Lentil and Sweet Potato Stew, 41

Lentil and Vegetable Soup, 46

M, N & O

Malfouf Salad (Lebanese Cabbage Salad), 113

No-Bake Blueberry Energy Bites, 87

Oatmeal with Berries and Flaxseed, 16

Oatmeal with Sliced Apples and Cinnamon, 32

P, Q & R

Pumpkin Oat Muffins, 90

Quinoa and Black Bean Bowl, 37

Quinoa and Black Bean Stuffed Peppers, 62

Quinoa and Chickpea Salad, 68

Quinoa and Vegetable Stir-Fry, 65

Quinoa Breakfast Bowl, 18

Quinoa Tabbouleh Salad, 109

Red Lentil and Carrot Soup, 55

Roasted Beet and Walnut Salad, 114

Roasted Chickpeas, 82

S

Sardine and Avocado Whole Grain Sandwich, 53

Seared Scallops with Spinach and Millet, 75

Shrimp and Vegetable Stir-Fry, 72

Smoothie with Spinach, Banana, and Flaxseed, 33

Spinach and Mushroom Omelette, 20

Spinach and Strawberry Salad, 118

Steamed Broccoli with Lemon-Garlic Dressing, 110

Stuffed Zucchini Boats, 67

Sweet Potato and Black Bean Hash, 28

Sweet Potato and Egg Hash, 19

T

Tempeh and Veggie Stir Fry, 57

Tofu Scramble, 27

Tofu Stir-Fry with Brown Rice, 52

Turkey and Avocado Wrap, 38

Turkey and Spinach Stuffed Bell Peppers, 51

Turmeric & Ginger Tea, 106

Turmeric & Pineapple Smoothie, 96

V

Vegetable and Tofu Stir-Fry, 31

Vegetable Breakfast Wrap, 23

Vegetable Buckwheat Bowl with Tahini Sauce, 76

W & Z

Warm Green Bean Salad, 115

Whole Grain Toast with Almond Butter and Banana, 30

Zucchini Noodles with Pesto and Cherry Tomatoes, 73

Printed in Dunstable, United Kingdom